Christmas 2000

To Jenny,

Celebrate who you are! A wonderful daughter, sister, friend, student, athlete and artist . . . and soon a Columbia co-ed!

Love,
Mommy & Daddy

I Am Beautiful™

A Celebration Of Women

EDITED BY

DANA CARPENTER & WOODY WINFREE

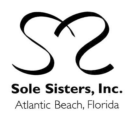

Sole Sisters, Inc.
Atlantic Beach, Florida

This work is lovingly dedicated to those who inspired us.

To my daughters, Layla and Romy.
May they always know their beauty.

— Woody Winfree

To the memory of my mother, Dorothy Dean,
and the future of my daughter, Kalie Dean.

— Dana Carpenter

First Printing, 1996: Rose Communications, L.L.C., Publisher

Cover and interior design: Tom Greensfelder, Nicole Ferentz and Brian Doyle

ISBN 0-9675113-0-5 (previously ISBN 1-887166-11-4)

Printed in the USA
Printing through Phelps & Associates, Lancaster, OH

To order *I Am Beautiful* directly from the publisher please call toll-free: 1-888-9BEAUTIFUL
Visit our website at **www.iambeautiful.com**
e-mail: ssisterinc@aol.com

ACKNOWLEDGMENTS

Our heartfelt thanks go to the many people who generously offered us their time and talents throughout the making of this book, to our family and friends who supported and guided us along the way, and to all the wonderfully courageous women who responded to our call. We offer special thanks to: Anonymous in St. Louis, David Bender, Pat Corrigan, Flavian Cresci, Mark Lawless, Elyse Shapiro and Deb Werksman.

Lastly, we give loving thanks to our husbands, Rick and Russell, for their tireless support and faith. We are grateful to be living our lives with partners who share so many of our beliefs and dreams.

Foreword

Above all else, this book was born out of the amazing friendship we share and our desire to illustrate for our daughters that all women can be embraced as beautiful, whole and worthy human beings.

Believing that a woman's sense of self-worth is inextricably linked to her sense of beauty, and that the images of beauty that surround us are narrow and often distorted, we wanted to effect change. As mothers guiding our own young daughters in a culture that puts too much emphasis on looks, we became committed to expanding the definition of beauty.

To do this, we knew we had to get the perspectives of as many women as possible. We went to real, everyday women like ourselves. "Tell us why you are beautiful," we requested. We placed ads in national magazines asking for photos and essays, created and mailed countless brochures, and spoke to interested reporters. Then we waited. We had no idea what we would hear back, if anything at all.

Slowly, responses started coming in from women across the country. In total, we received close to 500 submissions. The women featured in this book, along with the many others who replied, exposed their hearts, minds and souls in their remarkably trusting and generous answers to our simple, yet difficult question. All of the stories spoke to some part of us; many exposed us to new ideas; and others acted as mirrors.

We found ourselves with a body of work far beyond what we had imagined. And in the process, we received an incredible gift: the realization that we can, indeed, change our culture.

A greatly expanded and more inclusive definition of beauty begins with individual self-acceptance. We trust that this book will encourage women of all ages to name their own, unique beauty, and let it radiate for all to experience. In so doing, we will build a world in which every woman can say, "I Am Beautiful."

Dana Carpenter and Woody Winfree

As I approached my 30th birthday,

my older — and beautiful by any standard — cousin, told me that I would enjoy my thirties. She said women in their thirties have a "knowing beauty." A knowing beauty. That phrase stuck with me. To me, it means a beauty born of life experiences, good and bad, taken with patience and humor. Beauty comes when you love and are loved and you know it and believe it.

My beauty is enhanced when I relax and am kind to myself; when I allow myself a Sunday afternoon nap or fresh flowers. Most of all, I am relieved that outer, physical beauty can be transcended. I think less about how I look; I'm too busy with life. I take care of myself, I feel good and that is enough.

Karen with her dog, Feather
Jackson, Mississippi

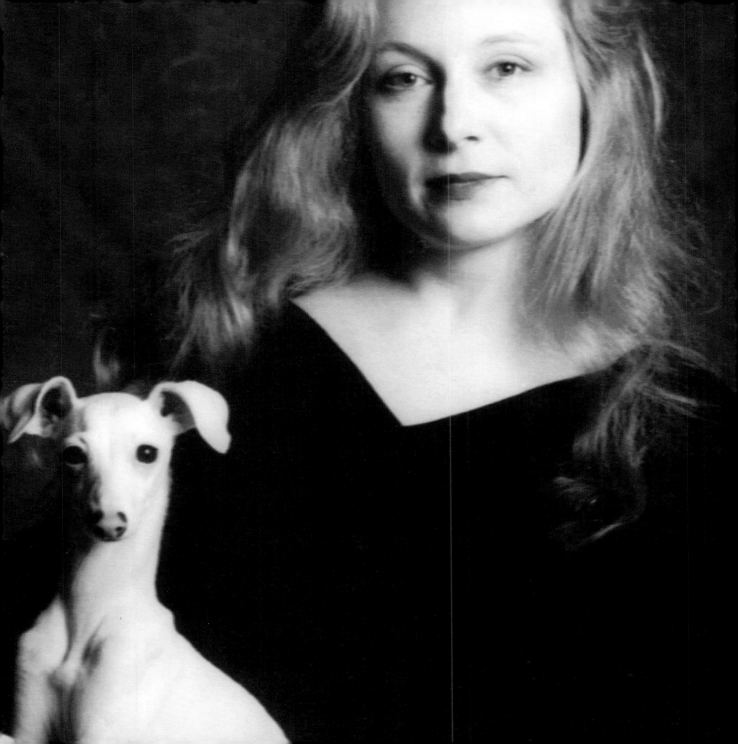

I WAS NEVER A BEAUTIFUL CHILD.

I was born during the Depression with a head full of matted black hair and it stayed that way for about eight years. My parents didn't pay much attention to what I looked like—survival was their priority.

When we had a few extra pennies I went to the barber shop with my uncles and got the same haircut as they got. The kids on the block teased me about whether I was a boy or a girl. Needless to say, I had an image problem that began in my youth, and I never felt beautiful.

Recently I encountered a familiar woman wheeling a baby carriage. She had been one of my son's playmates twenty years ago. She reminded me of one Christmas when I had been baking cookies. She had asked me why I had bothered to put an icing heart on one of the cookies that had come out crooked, why I hadn't thrown it away. I had instinctively answered: "Because we should love things that are not perfect."

She told me of how she thought of my words when her newborn son was brought to her with a deformity. Then she kissed me. Now whenever I look in the mirror, no matter what I see I think of her and her son, and know I am beautiful.

Joy
Golden's Bridge, New York

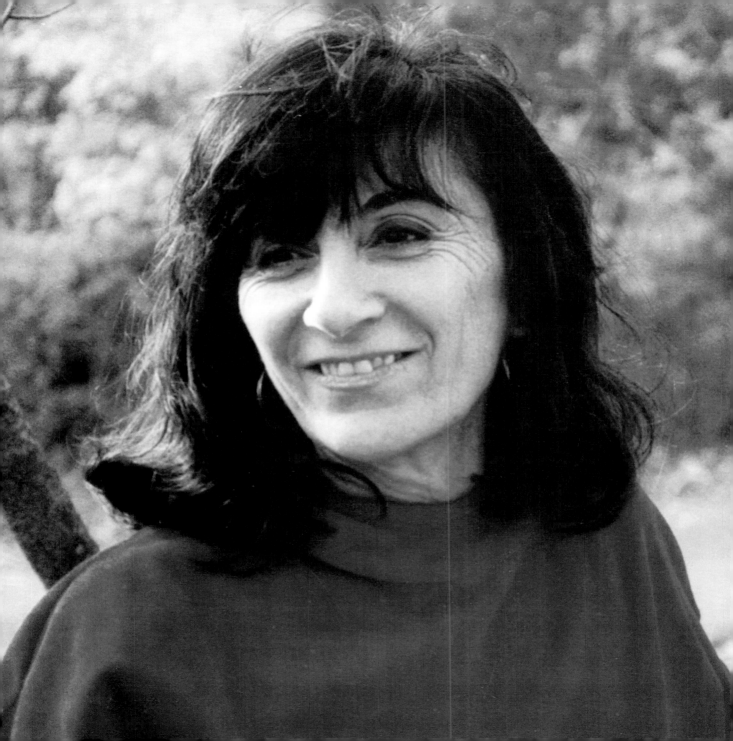

My Life is Full of Ah-Hahs.

Born during the hottest part of seventy summers ago
nurtured in a mother's love
anchored by a father's strength
adventured in childhood joys
searched for identity
traveled abroad
yearned for Mr. Right
married
mothered a darling baby
grieved her early death
suffered the pain, weathered the agony
and now
having a love affair with life!

Bee Jay
Prairie View, Texas

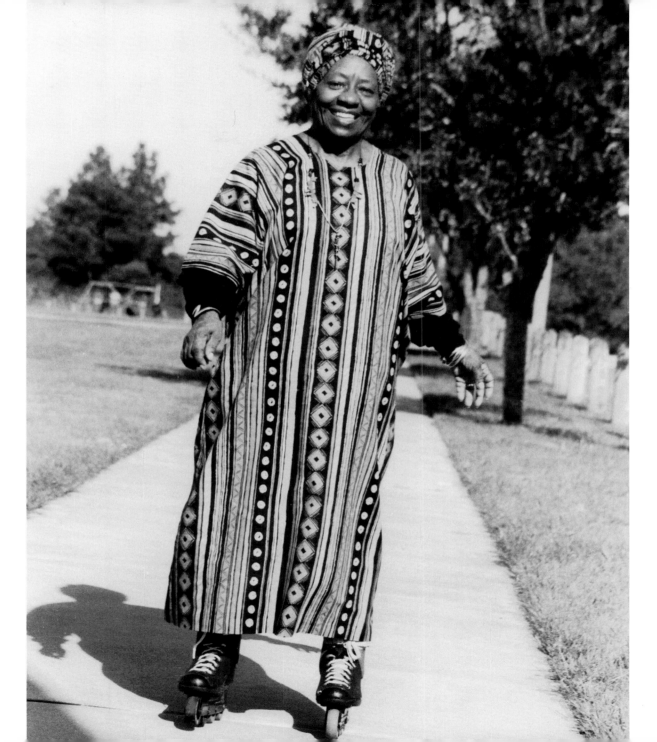

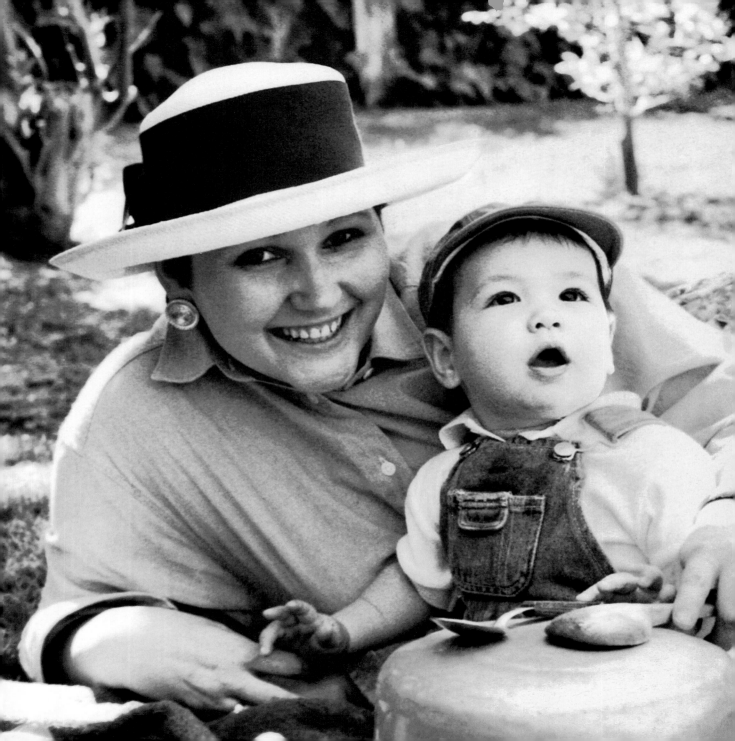

THE BEAUTY OF MY BODY

is not measured by the size of the clothes it can fit into, but by the stories that it tells. I have a belly and hips that say, "We grew a child in here," and breasts that say, "We nourished life." My hands, with bitten nails and a writer's callous, say, "We create amazing things."

Sarah with her son, Nathaniel
Glencoe, Illinois

THE JOY OF MAKING AND SHARING MUSIC

with others is the source of the beauty that comes from within me. In 75 years, my life has taken many turns. I have known the thrill of watching fresh young faces smile through their first recitals, and the sense of accomplishment when a student of mine becomes a teacher. I have experienced the utter heartbreak that death brings with the passing of my parents, my husband, and most recently, the loss of my son to AIDS. At each turn, the piano has been a constant friend, my strength. It has sustained and comforted me. It has touched my life, and through it, I have touched the lives of many around me.

Marjorie
Jacksonville Beach, Florida

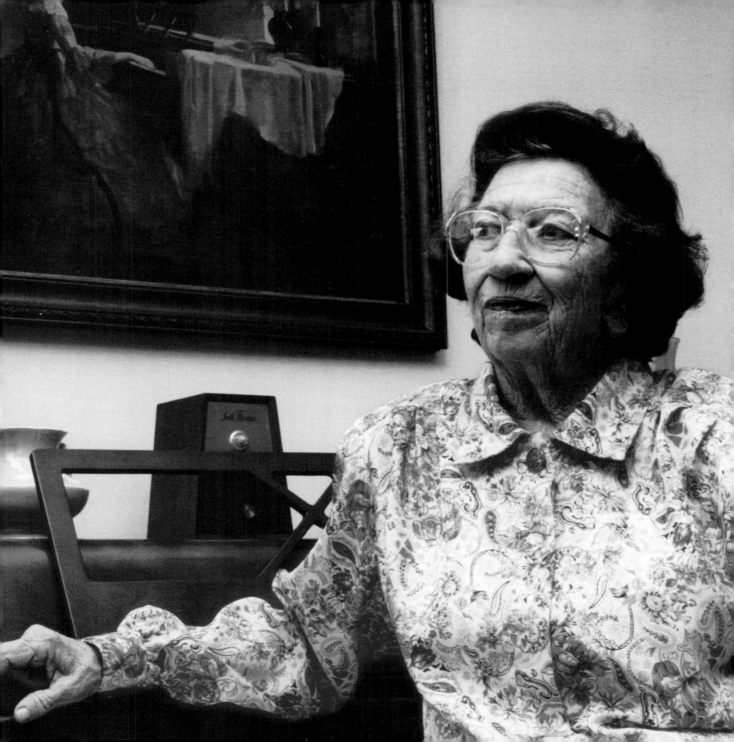

I AM FULL OF WONDER AND IDEAS,

and I think this energy surrounds me. Despite the chronic physical pain that I live with, my friends see a radiance in me. Their ability to see this radiance, their friendships, feed my happiness. And for the moments we are together, it eclipses my pain.

zana
Tucson, Arizona

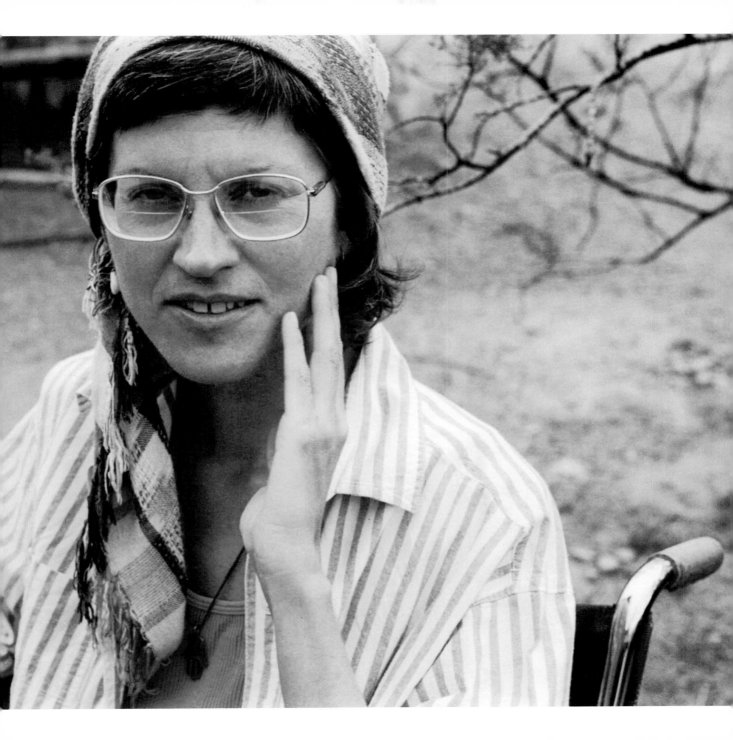

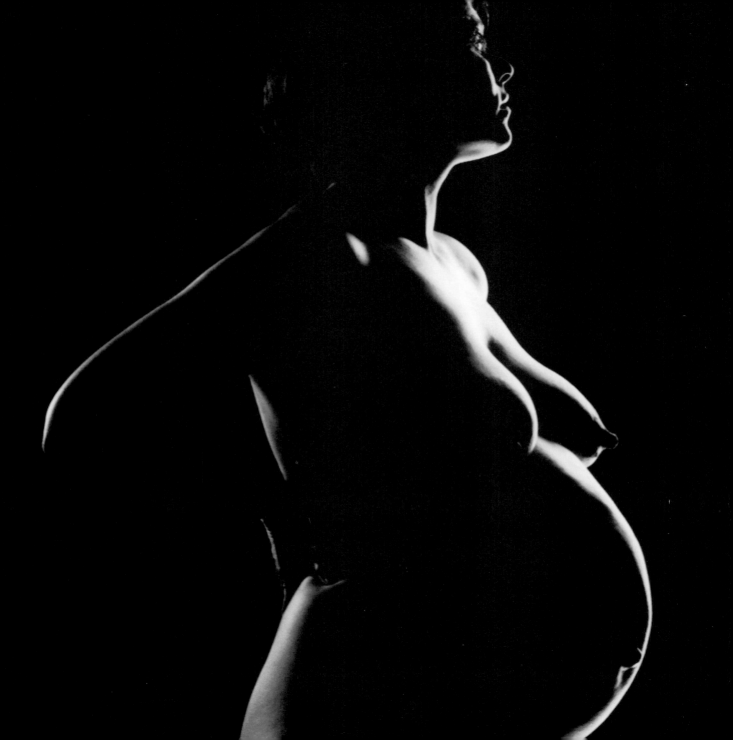

I LOVE EVERY CURVE OF MY SILKY FLESH.

Shoulder, breast, belly, thigh—this roundness is surely the shape that I was meant to be. At forty years old, carrying my fourth child, I feel strong and sensuous, my juices flowing freely. I cherish this last chance of glowing in the round. I am a full moon, the Goddess incarnate.

Susan
Victoria, British Columbia

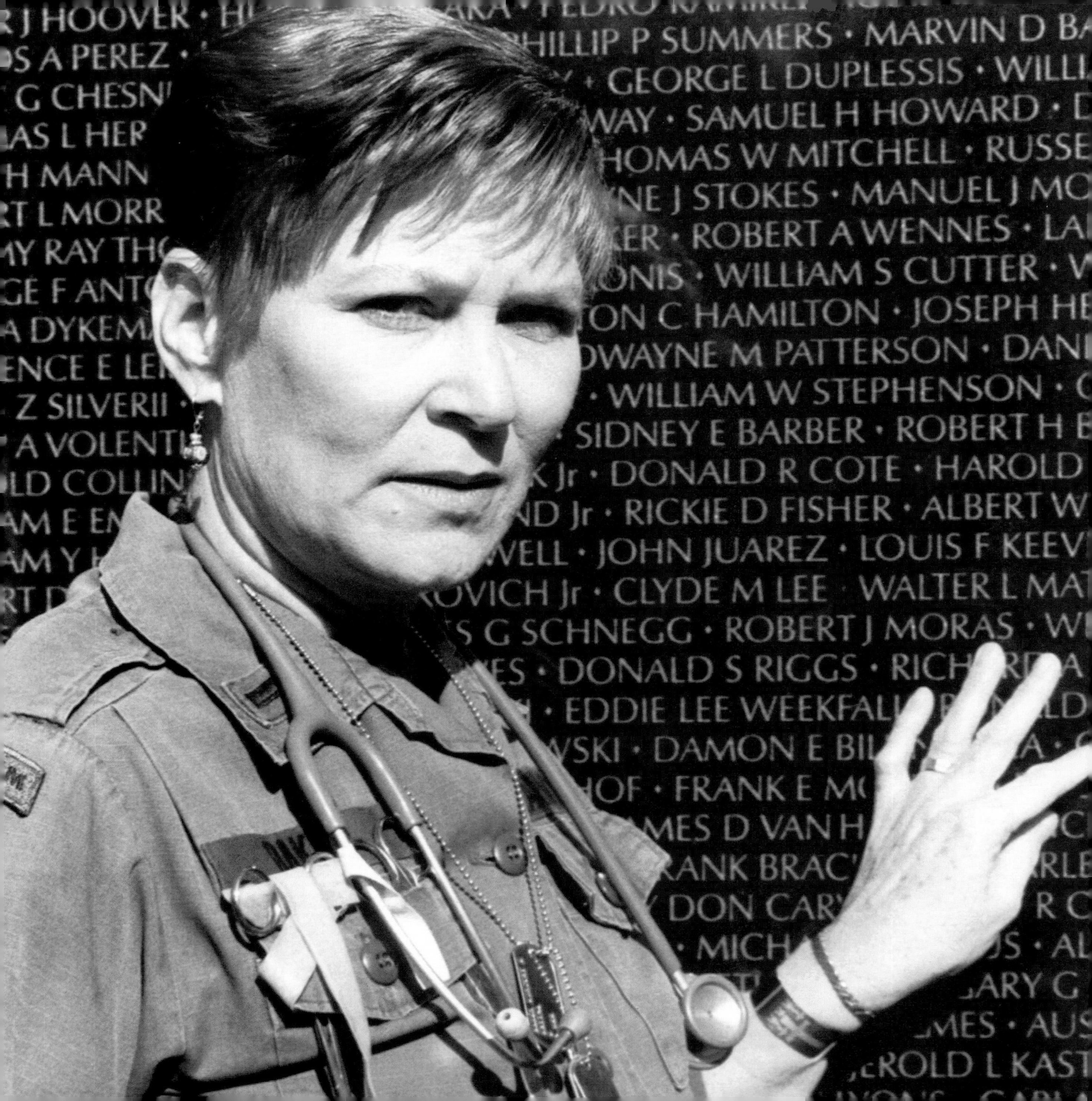
GEORGE L DUPLESSIS
SAMUEL H HOWARD
ROBERT A WENNES
WILLIAM S CUTTER
DWAYNE M PATTERSON
WILLIAM W STEPHENSON
SIDNEY E BARBER
DONALD R COTE
RICKIE D FISHER
JOHN JUAREZ
CLYDE M LEE
ROBERT J MORAS
DONALD S RIGGS

TRY AS I MIGHT,

I am not able to say anything about beauty that is more meaningful to me than the few lines I wrote nearly three decades ago as a twenty-year-old Army nurse in Vietnam:

Like swans on still water they skim
    over the war
Ao dais gliding, rustling serenely
gleaming black hair pulled primly away
from faces that reveal nothing
    save inner repose,
a beauty so deep even war can't defile.

I note my reflection in their obsidian eyes
an outsized barbarian, ungainly, unkempt,
baggy in ever-wilted greens,
five-pound boots taking plowhand strides,
face perpetually ruddy, dripping in alien heat.

In their delicate presence I exhume
    teenage failures
the girl in the back row forever unnoticed,
the one no one ever invited to dance,
the one never voted most-likely anything,

the one who was never quite
    something enough.

But once in a while, on a crazy-shift morning,
when I've worked through the night
    and I'm too tired to care,
a young man who reeks of rice paddies
    lies waiting
for someone to heal the new hole in his life.
He says through his pain, all adolescent
    bravado,
"Hey, what's your name? Let's get married.
    I love you."

And just for a moment I become Nefertiti
and for all the Orient's pearls and silks
I would not trade the glamour and privilege
of these honored hands, licensed to touch
    one filthy GI.

Dana
Chicago, Illinois

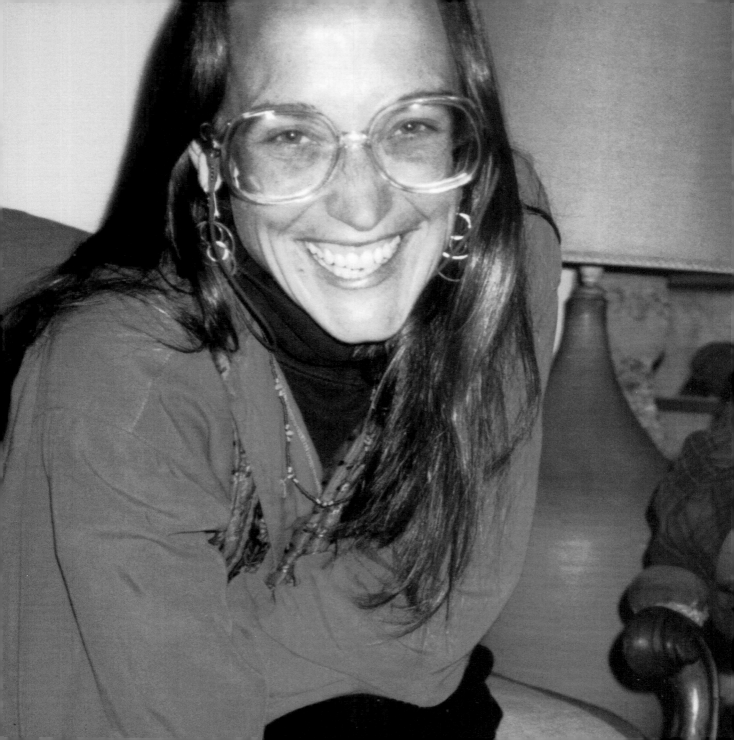

HIDING BEHIND THICK GLASS

to hold off hurt,
a little girl
wishes
to see no more

She cannot know
the fragile barrier
she creates
will only invite
new pain

Vulnerable now
to the ridicule
of siblings,
the impermanence
of glass and plastic
held together by pins

She succumbs
to the isolation
imposed
and denies

she was
ever
beautiful

Modern medicine
redeems
her teenage years
Her new secret;
the lenses
she wears
for the next two decades

At thirty-six
while on holiday
the contact slips
the spiral turns

she must face
herself
as a
wearing glasses woman

A picture taken
brings shock
and revelation—
a beautiful woman
laughs
at the camera

Joyful woman
leaning forward woman
claiming her space woman

Alive, glistening with
    health woman
wearing glasses woman
beautiful woman

Ní Aódagaín
Waldport, Oregon

WHEN I WAS YOUNG

I was indeed a beauty—tall, slender, striking. What a pity I never enjoyed it. A childhood with a vain, self-occupied mother did nothing to reassure me and I never saw myself as beautiful. It never occurred to me that people on the street who turned and stared were admiring my beauty. I always assumed that they saw a freak—too tall, too thin, too conspicuous. It wasn't until that beauty slipped away—the jaw line not so clean, the eyes puffy, the lines developing around the mouth—that I began to look at old photos and think, "My word, I was a beauty, wasn't I!"

Now I am sixty. But I am more beautiful than the gorgeous creature who struggled unenlightened through the earlier years.

I have forgiven my mother.

I have survived unemployment, divorce, single-parenthood, and cancer.

I am quiet, all restlessness spent. Anger no longer fills the nooks and crannies of my soul.

I am content to accept the present and what is good in it—enough to eat, a roof, so many books to read, so much music to hear, gifts to give.

I take nothing for granted—the feel of clean sheets against my skin, the gentle onset of sleep, the smell of freshly cut grass, the kindness of friends.

I have come to accept my solitary life as what is truly best for me.

I know that I have occupied my little space and time on earth, breathed my little bit of air.

I have seen my genes marching into the future on sturdy little legs.

I have made my inward journey—and found myself.

Adilee with her granddaughter, Gracie
New Castle, Delaware

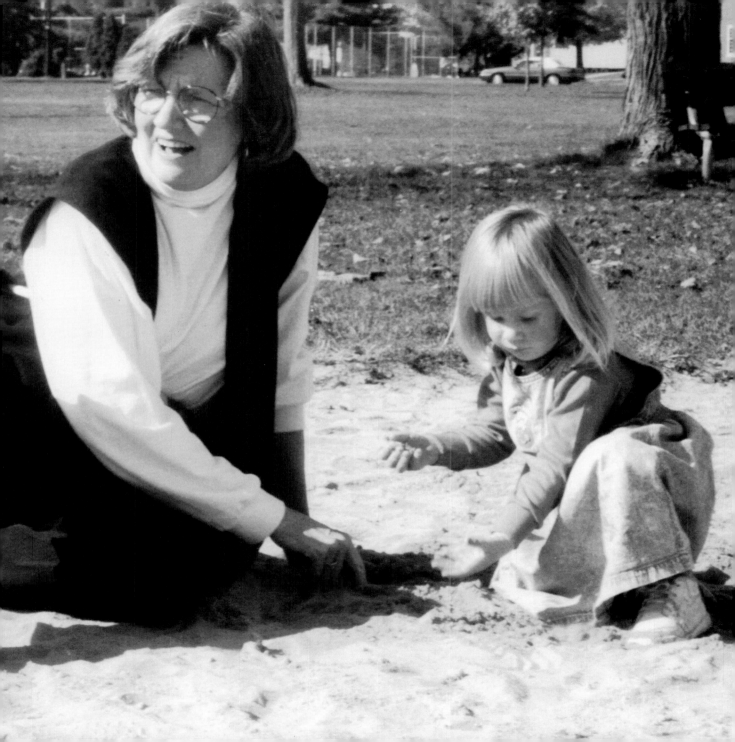

I ENTER MY MID-TWENTIES

a single woman and well-meaning friends and family are showing their concern. Although I have a college degree, have traveled around the world, and love my job working with children, I am still an "unmarried woman."

I hope to marry and have children, but I refuse to wait around for someone to save me from the big, bad world. Instead of being encouraged to live my life to the fullest, with or without a partner, I sometimes feel like I have an expiration date on my forehead.

Sure, I've lapsed into temporary fits of panic as my collection of bridesmaid dresses grows. Then I remember all the things I've learned the past few years, and how I needed time by myself to learn the true meaning of self-reliance. I won't be young forever, but my appreciation for life and the confidence I've gained will keep me feeling beautiful for the rest of my life.

Hilary
Houston, Texas

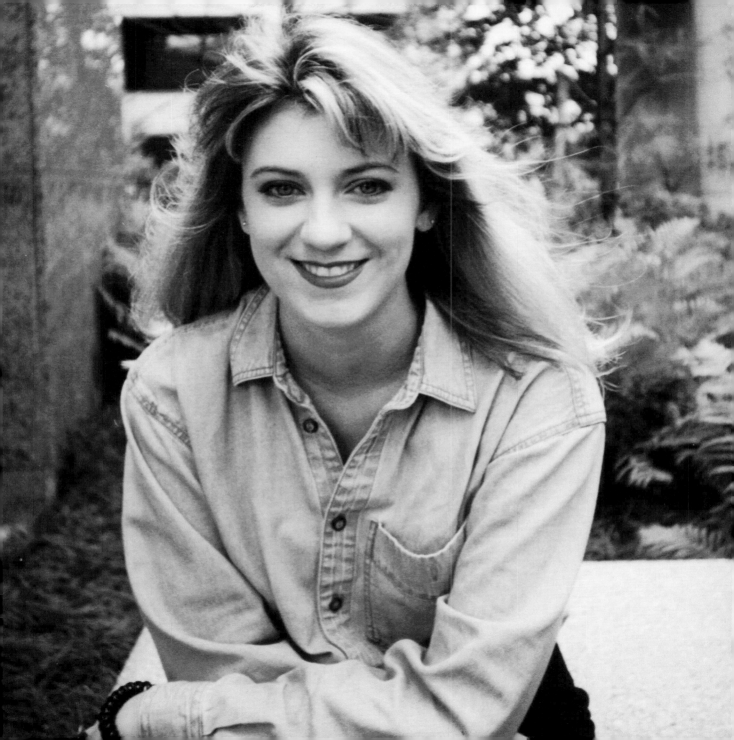

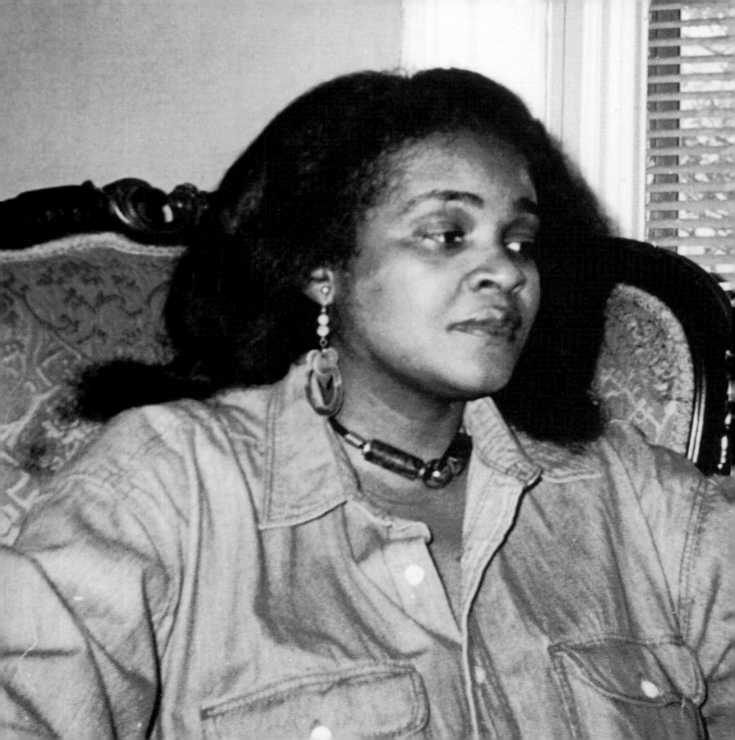

NAMELESS, LONG DEAD,

remembered only for
her color.

Black like molasses,
tar, ink, coal.
So black she absorbed
    everything around her.
Midnight had wrapped itself
    around this woman.
They said she had looks
    to match that black
    skin of hers.
She was strong with
    that beauty.
She was my mother.
I reflect her.

Mother of my kinky hair,
wide hips,
and big legs.

She was a native woman—
Brown like honey—
Round like skillet cornbread.
They said she told stories
that made you laugh.

Mother of my long legs,
Black hair,
Height like a tree.
She was the one who
    taught me
her cooking secrets in
    my sleep.

She was bold and fearless
with her looks.
She was the
mother of pleasure,
laughter, and fun.

I am beautiful because
I carry
beauty deep
in blood and bone.
Nameless women, ancestors
    of mine,
gave me gifts
of color,
humor,
and a magic touch
with pots and pans.
They are my mothers.
I reflect them.

Pat
Richmond, Indiana

I THOUGHT BEAUTY MEANT YOU WERE THIN,

So I began a game that no one wins.

At my ninth birthday I ate no cake,
By ten all that mattered was my weight.

One, two, seven years passed by,
While I counted calories and slowly died.

Grade school and junior high were finished,
In the yearbook I was voted slimmest.

My world came to a halt in high school,
I finally realized anorexia was not cool.

Recovery was slow, setbacks were rough,
Accepting a new body was certainly tough.

But I am better, I've beaten this disease,
And now I know what beauty means.

I thought it meant you had to be thin,
But in truth, beauty lies beyond one's skin.

What makes me beautiful, what do I say?
It is who I am, not that I look a certain way.
I am beautiful because I understand children
        and we make each other smile;
I am beautiful because I help other people;
I am beautiful because I have a love for life;
I am beautiful because I care about
        our world;

I am beautiful because I am me.

Karen
Fox Point, Wisconsin

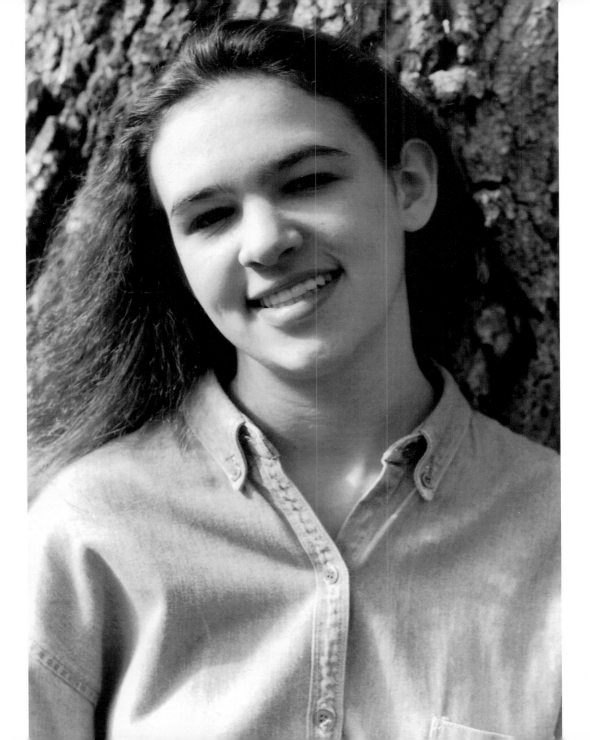

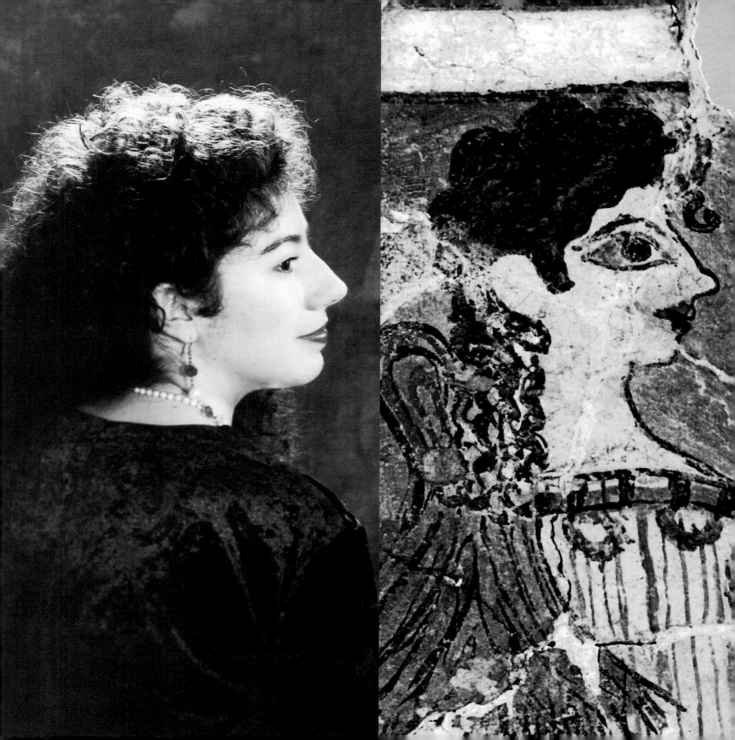

THE REMARKABLE RESEMBLANCE

between the Minoan priestess's distinct profile and my own strikes me deeply. It is a great, magical affirmation of my beauty, strength, and connection to our ancient feminine heritage. It makes me think I must have had past lives as a priestess in which I stood proud, confident, empowered. It affirms the importance of my spiritual path in this lifetime to assist humanity in embracing and reintegrating the feminine once more. It helps me heal from the sadness I've felt over not measuring up to the image of button-nosed, blonde-haired, blue-eyed beauty so prized by our culture. It reassures me that my rich, exotic looks make me glorious, too.

Marguerite
Cambridge, Massachusetts

WIDE HIPS AND ALL,

I celebrate my newly acquired Goddessness. There was a time when I didn't think I had it in me to be womanly. How many voices had I heard say, "Big women can't be attractive or feminine." And for awhile I believed, turning to drugs and alcohol to maintain a smaller, more acceptable figure.

Now, at 34, I have come to the conclusion that this is the me that I am meant to be. Barely 5' 3" with short-cropped hair and *café con leche* skin, everything about me proudly shouts "Unconventional!" Full of life and love, I sing the praises of lovely women everywhere — I share our beauty.

Dineta
Palm Springs, California

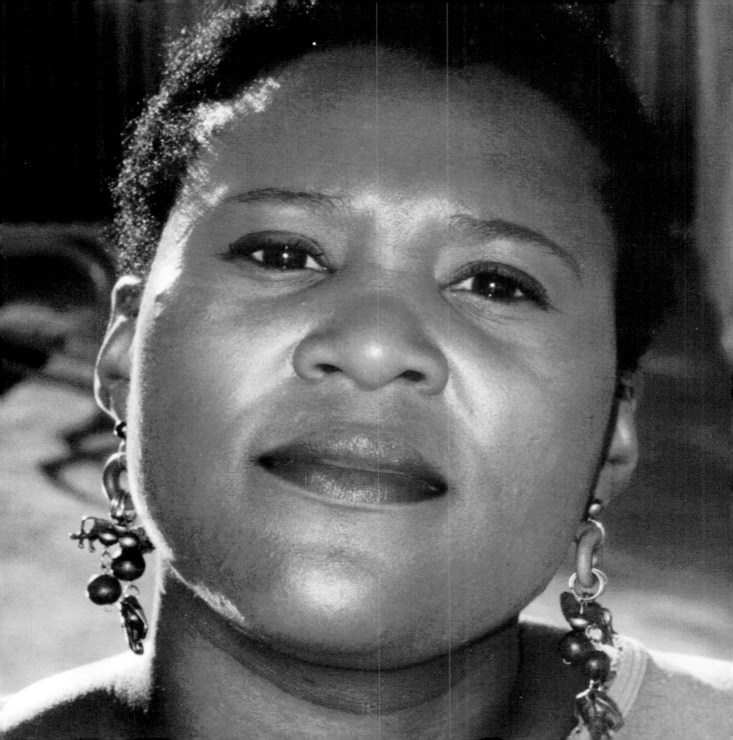

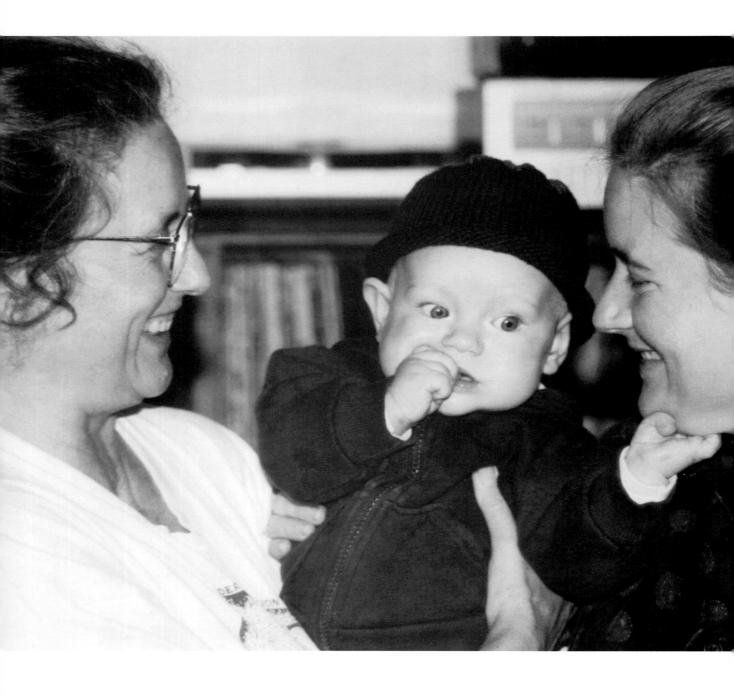

I AM BEAUTIFUL, ESPECIALLY

because I chose the long, hard journey of breaking my family's destructive pattern: young, unmothered mothers being hard on their daughters. I passed on far more of the hurt than I ever wanted to, but I realized early enough that the road of repair led straight through my own mothering. I have three daughters and a son, and now a first granddaughter. I see more and more how the process begun years ago has worked slowly over time, like nature. And much of the beauty, healing, and health will manifest in generations beyond my time. The joy of relating to my children in the present—the joy of being with my first daughter as she gave birth to her first daughter—is beyond measure. My family is connected. We are beautiful.

Oosa with her granddaughter, Chiara,
and her daughter, Kelcey
Cazadero, California

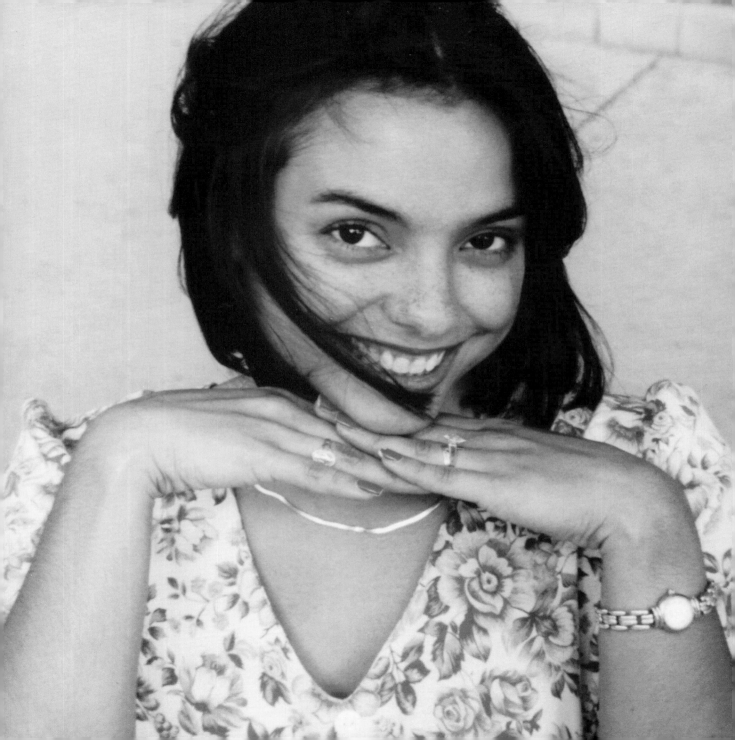

WHEN I STARTED STRIPPING, I FELT BEAUTIFUL.

At nineteen years old, I was insecure and struggling through college. Taking that job changed everything in my life—into a circus of errors and delusion. While salty men stared lecherously at my naked body, somehow I felt beautiful. "All these men want me, so I must be good," I thought.

I tried to ignore the fact that I was being abused. My drinking got severely out of hand. Days went by that I couldn't remember. School became a nuisance. My mother quit talking to me, and I didn't care.

One day I hit a brick wall. All of a sudden I knew that I was dying inside. I looked in the mirror and saw the remnants of a trampled flower. Tired, wilted, I gave it all up.

The same day I told my employer to get lost, I buried the bottle for good. After avoiding myself for three years, I became my own best friend. At 23, I am just learning to love myself. And finally, with a few extra layers of clothing and self-respect, I know I am beautiful.

Kay
Chicago, Illinois

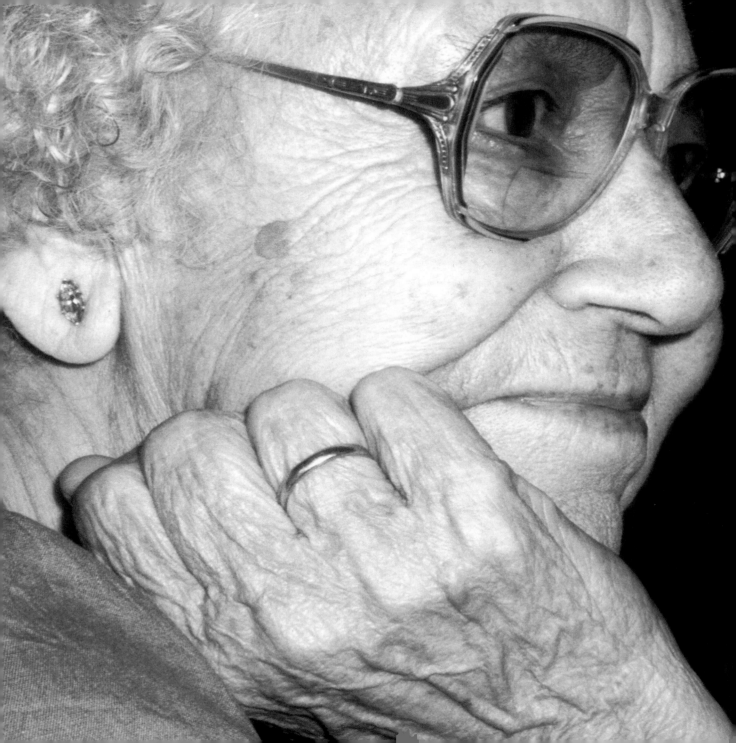

I'M AN OLD LADY, WRINKLED AND GRAY.

But beauty, it comes from the inside.
I love people and I got a good nature.
So, yes, maybe I am beautiful.

Judith
New Port Richey, Florida

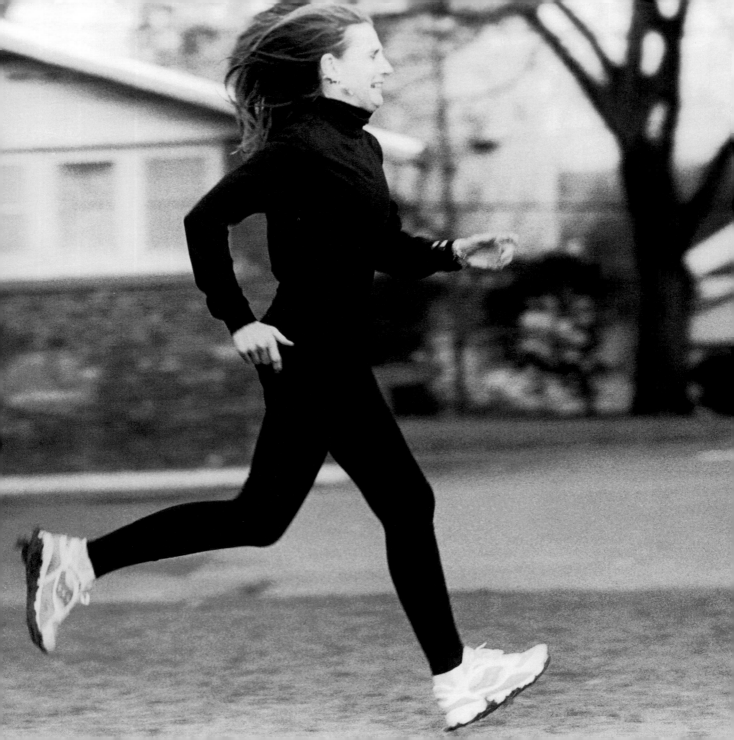

I AM STRONG.

I started running about six months ago and already I've run in several races—including my first half-marathon.
A few years from now, when I am 50, I want to do a triathlon.

I am sensual.
I celebrate my sexuality. I love sex. I'm tender and loving.
I hold my children, my lover. I hug my friends. I love my students.

I am smart.
My family and teachers had no faith in my scholastic abilities. They said I would never be able to finish school. Two degrees later, rich with self-taught skills—from photography to roofing—I celebrate the power and richness of my mind.

Maureen
Portland, Oregon

IN MY YOUTH, I WAS TAUGHT

that a beautiful woman has the facial features of Elizabeth Taylor, the body of Marilyn Monroe, and the class of Grace Kelly. That she must be demure, charming and not terribly bright.

At 52, I cling to that image, although intellectually, I know that beauty is abstract and individually defined.

I struggle even to write this, and yet, in the last few years I have come to understand that I am a physically attractive woman who holds a powerful job and who applies that power in a judicious manner. I have come to understand that it's okay to be smart, creative, and assertive, wear short hair, have a flat chest, and walk like a duck.

Lynne with her dog, Rosie
Fresno, California

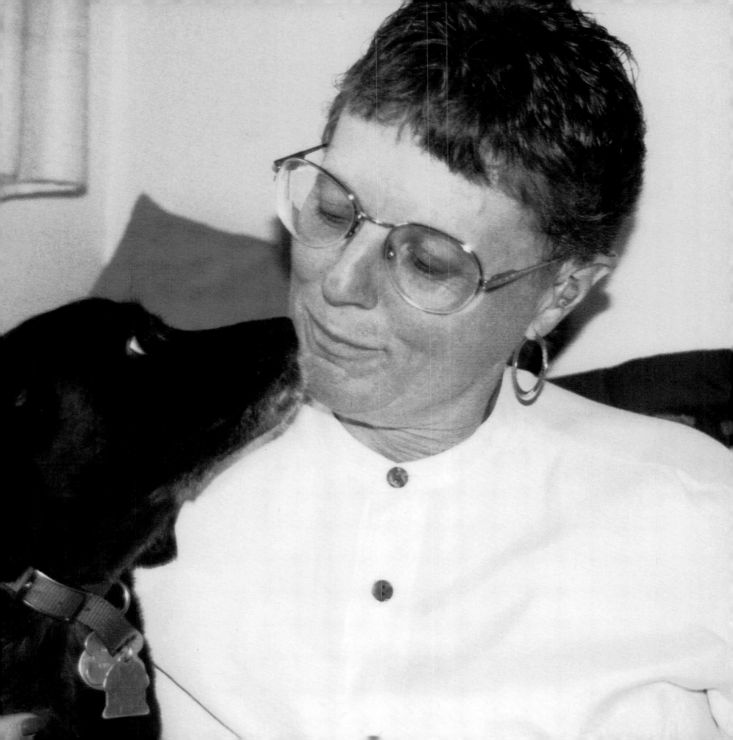

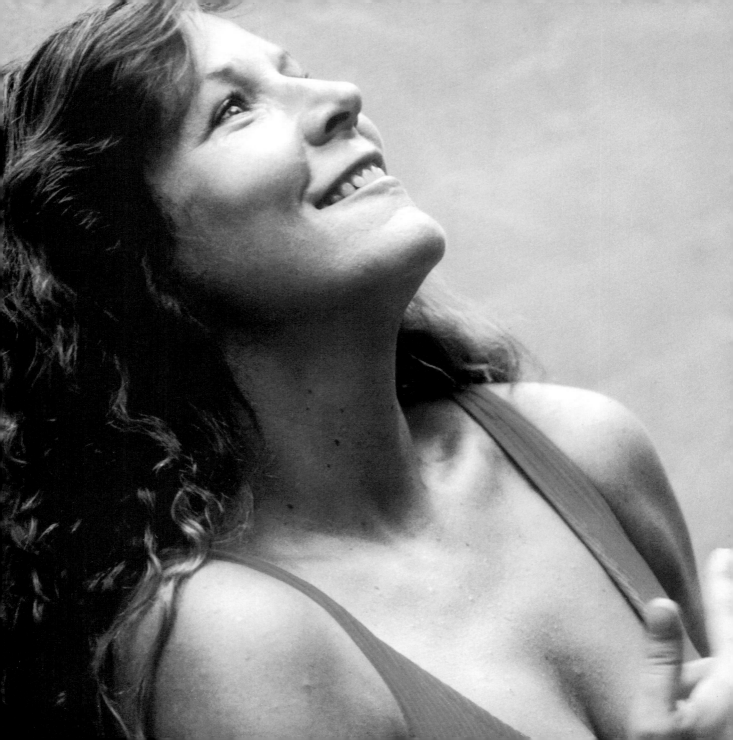

I AM REDISCOVERING

the radiant child I was long ago; this is where my beauty lies. Once a spontaneous, cheerful, and curious babe, I lost these attributes with my innocence as the result of sexual abuse. Along with self-esteem issues due to this abuse, I was taunted and teased as a child about my size. Being as strong and strapping as the boys my age was an asset when being chosen for team sports, but not when being chosen for dates.

With time, my wide-eyed wonder has returned and I have come to see myself as an attractive woman. I am a vibrant, 36-year-old, 5'10", full-figured, big-boned gal of Ukrainian and Irish heritage. I am beautiful because I like who I am.

Tamara Joy
Tucson, Arizona

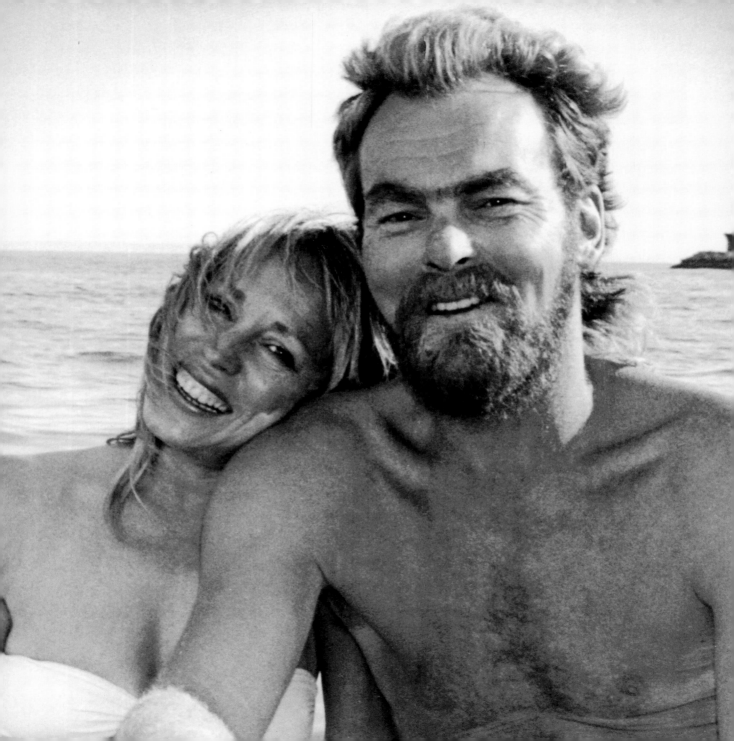

BEAUTIFUL IS POSING

for your wedding invitation
with your best friend of 25 years.

Claire with her husband, Kevin
Rowayton, Connecticut

I AM A RECOVERING DRUG ADDICT.

It's been 12 years since I quit.

As an addict, I was on my way to killing myself. I didn't think I deserved to live.

I felt unworthy—a feeling that started in childhood as a result of emotional abuse.

In the last 12 years, I have gone through a lot of emotional and spiritual healing.

About 5 years ago, when I was 36, I decided to live out my dream of being a jazz singer.

I worked very hard at it, and in 1994 I was chosen to sing in the Chicago Jazz Festival.

I feel I am proof that God does help those who help themselves. I have become a very honest, responsible, and productive member of society—I work as a court reporter in Chicago. My whole life has changed through hard work, help from others, and God.

I'm very grateful to be alive and able to live my dreams. I love who I am today. I have a beautiful life.

Hinda
Chicago, Illinois

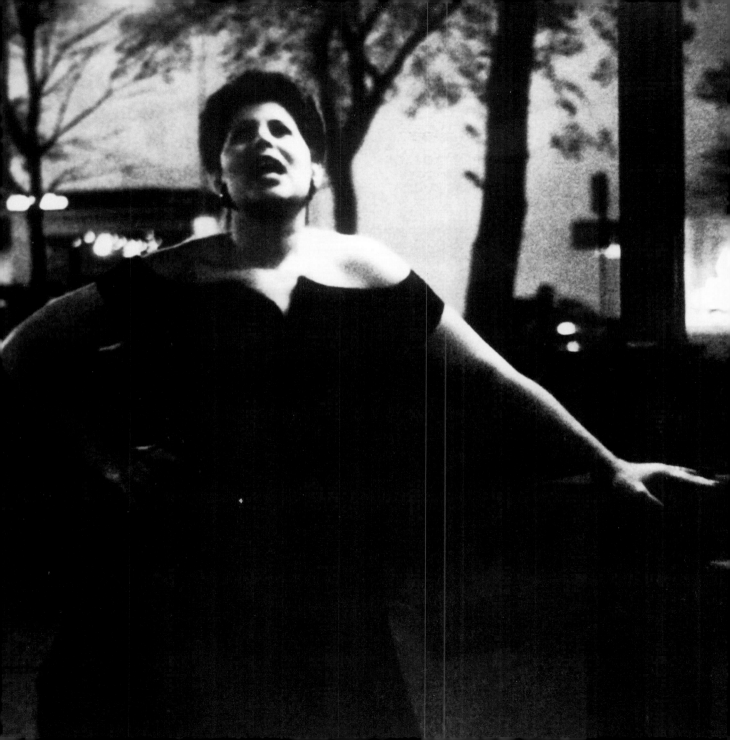

I AM MOST BEAUTIFUL WHEN

I am happy, so here I am on a whale-watching tour. The wonderful glow you see is the result of my doing something fun and exciting. Not only did I learn a lot through this experience, I believe the people with me learned something too. I tried to show them, especially the children, that fat people can do lots of things as long as they are healthy. Plus, I told them, we have the advantage of an extra layer to keep us warm. . .

Mary
Santa Cruz, California

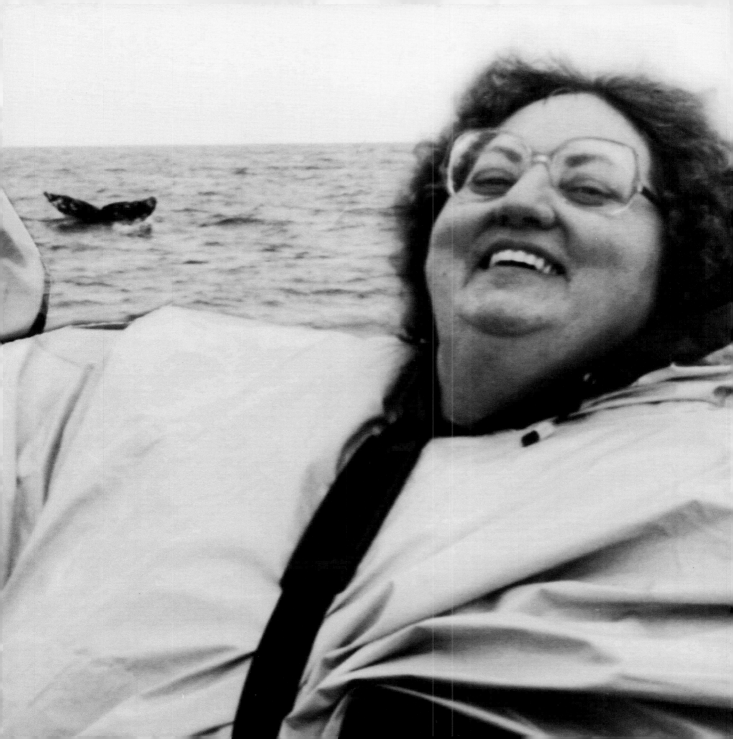

LOOK AT ME!

I am one of the beautiful people—37 and slightly fantastic.

My long, slender neck holds a remarkable face, which shows plenty of character. Crinkles of enhancement circle my green twinkling eyes. Lines of laughter and mischief surround an inviting smile. High cheekbones highlight and accentuate my strong, but feminine nose. My thin lips, cleft chin, and the space between my top front teeth are distinctive and add to my otherwise perfect features.

The rest of me is heavenly. Just ask my husband, he'll tell you. I am beautiful inside and out!

Debi
Saugus, Massachusetts

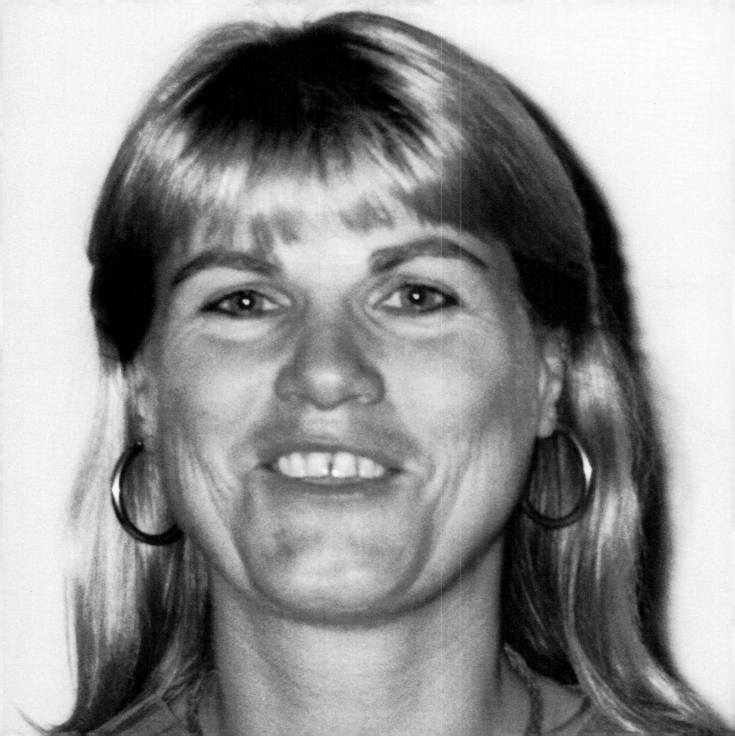

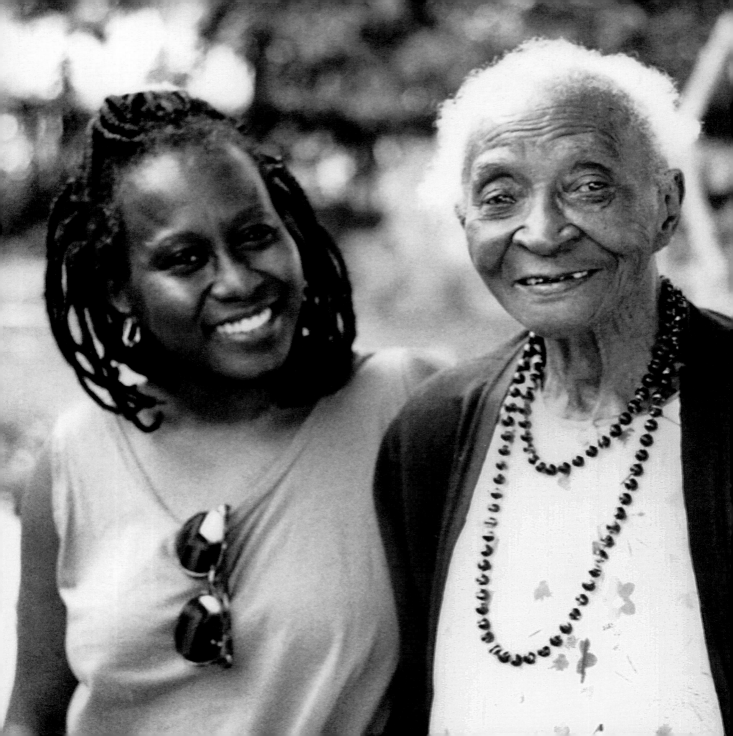

Growing up in Jamaica,

my beauty was pointed out at every turn by women in my community. My mother was beautiful and everyone said I looked like her. By the time I was 3 years old my beauty was something I took for granted. However, as I grew older, I learned that beauty did not merely refer to facial or physical features, and could be enhanced by a friendly, easy-going disposition. Like my mother, I enjoyed laughter. You could say laughter found us in every corner and at all times. Since this laughter, and love, were a reflection of the community from which I came, I have never doubted my beauty.

Opal with her grandmother, Edith
Oakland, California

63 YEARS MY BODY AND I HAVE BEEN TOGETHER.

It has climbed a lot of trees, hung upside down on monkey bars, and pumped swings high up to the sky. I like the expression I see in the mirror; it's still familiar even though it has relaxed a bit and it is wearing age spots where freckles once were.

My long arms have spiked volleyballs, my long legs have wrapped around horses' bellies, bareback. In my strong body, two babies have floated in utero, split the ring, suckled my bursting breasts, and sagged in my aching arms.

My deft fingers, which once spread watercolor on more than two thousand original paintings, now fly over the keyboard of my computer, recording fairy tales complete with illustrations. My mind cooperates in this new job, even though my eyes are playing hide and seek.

My juicy, elegant, playful, beautiful body and I are still happy in each other's company.

Ruth
Gualala, California

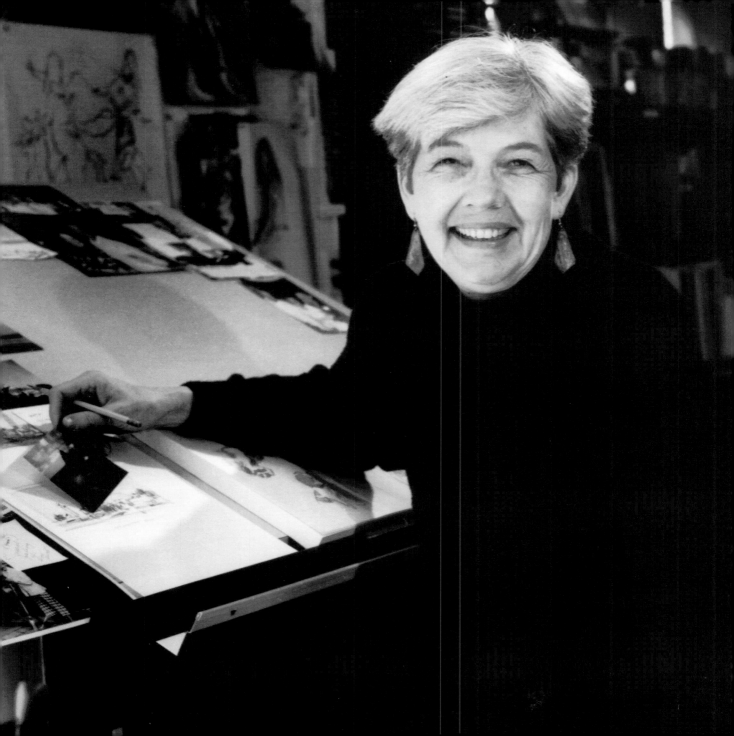

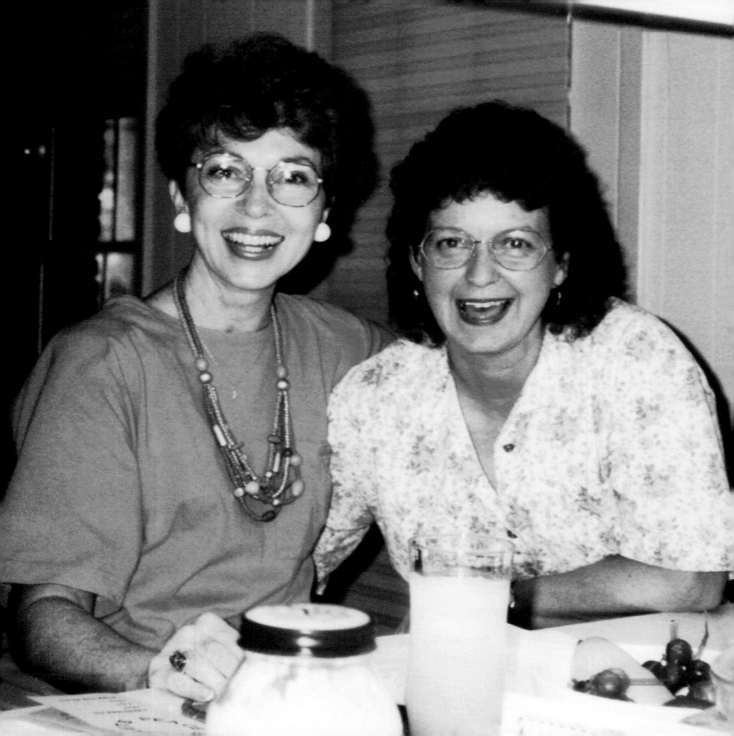

FRIENDS.
WE STARTED ON A SEARCH FOR BEAUTY

together 20 years ago. We found beauty in each other's eyes and in the support and strength of a friendship which was nurtured through the illnesses and deaths of our parents, the slow recovery of a drug-addicted teenager, the rejection of another, cancer, and the geographical separation of oceans.

Strength of spirit emerged through tears, prayers, encouragement, gentle admonition, and countless cups of tea.

Our adult daughters haven't missed seeing the beauty we have. They share their wishes of obtaining the richness of a friendship like ours. And so we have arrived at the mid-point of our life journey. We asked our husbands to snap this picture because we are proud of how "smart" we look in our new bifocals.

Susan and Linda
Clinton, Mississippi and Vienna, Virginia

I HAVE LOST ALL OF MY HAIR

to chemotherapy, yet my husband tells me every day that I am beautiful. The look in his eyes tells me that he really sees me as beautiful. When the pain is too great to sleep at night, he holds me close. I sense his deep love for me and that makes the pain bearable.

I have been told that inoperable ovarian cancer gives me six months to a year to live. I don't accept this, and have found that I have an inner strength to fight. This has helped me to realize that the beauty my husband sees does not lie in hair, makeup, or a perfect "10" figure. It comes from the peace that I feel within.

Jean
Ft. Collins, Colorado

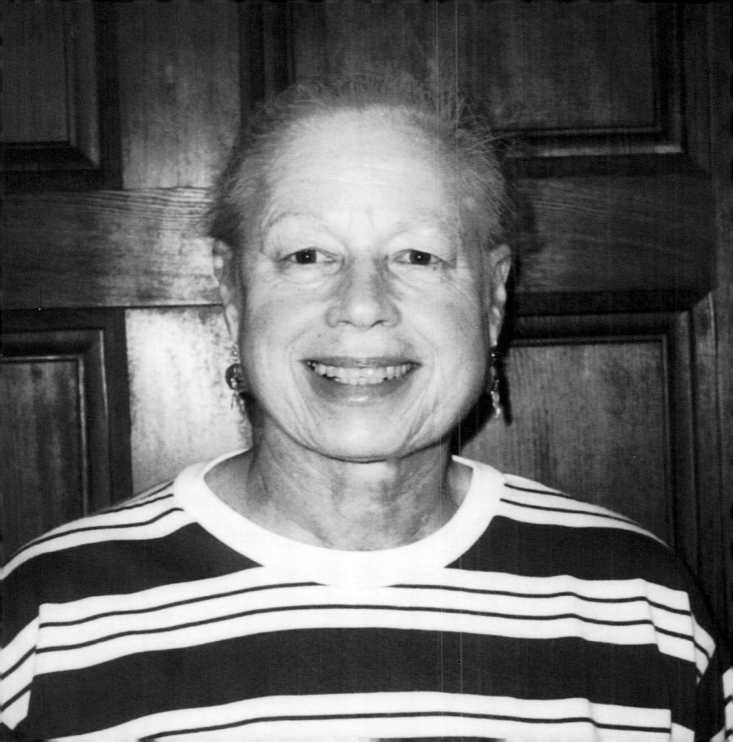

I QUIT THE PH. D. PROGRAM.

I no longer needed others to validate my intelligence or my scholarship.

The act was beautiful: original, unexpected, and unique.

I was beautiful: assertive, proud, forceful, and angry.

Perhaps I waited half a lifetime to show real emotion, an authentic response to something deeply felt. Anger. Anger at the missed opportunity to reveal what I knew.

I quit the conformity, endless jockeying, mind games and mind-sets, posturing, groveling, and servile dependence.

In an academic discipline with no room for discussion and doubt, freedom and openness, I was choking.

To exhibit deeply felt emotion in all its nakedness is real beauty.

The emotion is mine, and I own it.

I am beautiful because of it.

Helen
Carbondale, Illinois

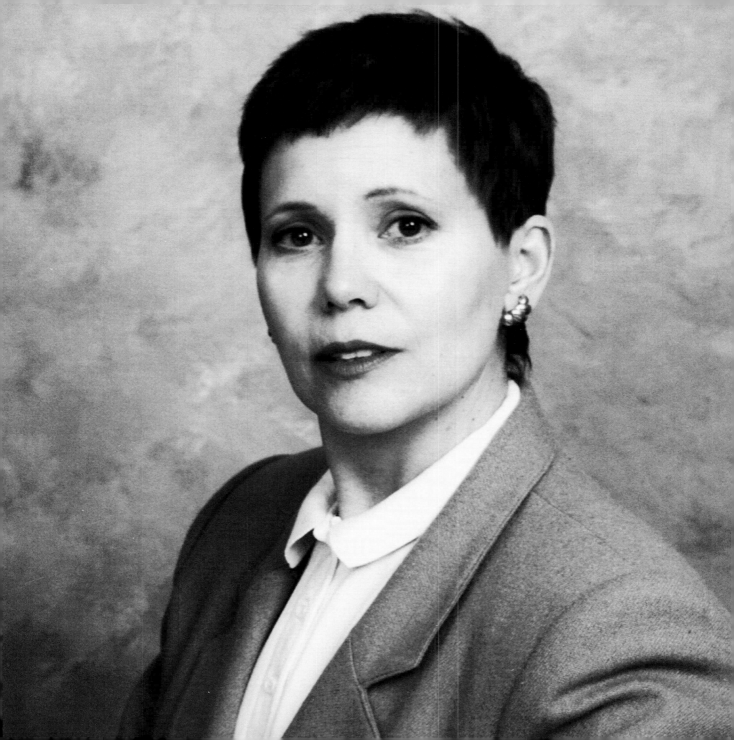

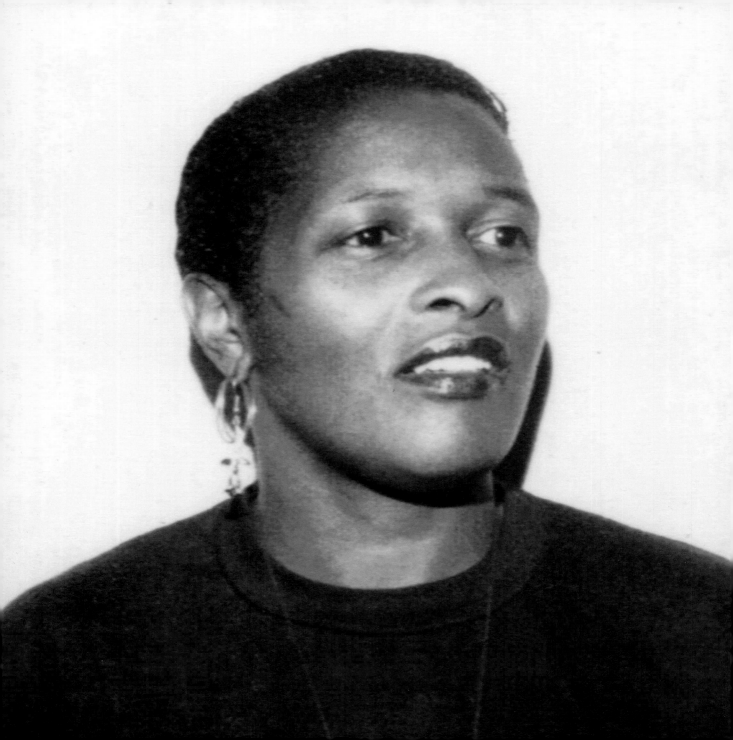

MY GOD-GIVEN BEAUTY

is not a physical attribute, but an insightful and empathetic manner of relating to both friends and strangers. People who are distressed seek me out. This has been true throughout my life. And as a telephone operator, I talk with a lot of people.

One morning a young man called, sobbing. He was threatening to kill himself. I talked to him for over 30 minutes: he told me his story; we cried and prayed together. I assured him that God loved him even though he felt so loveless. Near the end of the conversation he repeatedly asked who I was, if I was an angel. He said I saved his life.

At that moment I knew that God had put me in touch with this person. I was elated. Before we closed, I got his number and made him promise that he wouldn't do anything to hurt himself or prevent him from answering the phone when I called back. When I got home I called him, he answered, and we cried some more.

God is beautiful and brings out the beauty in me.

Verna
Williamstown, New Jersey

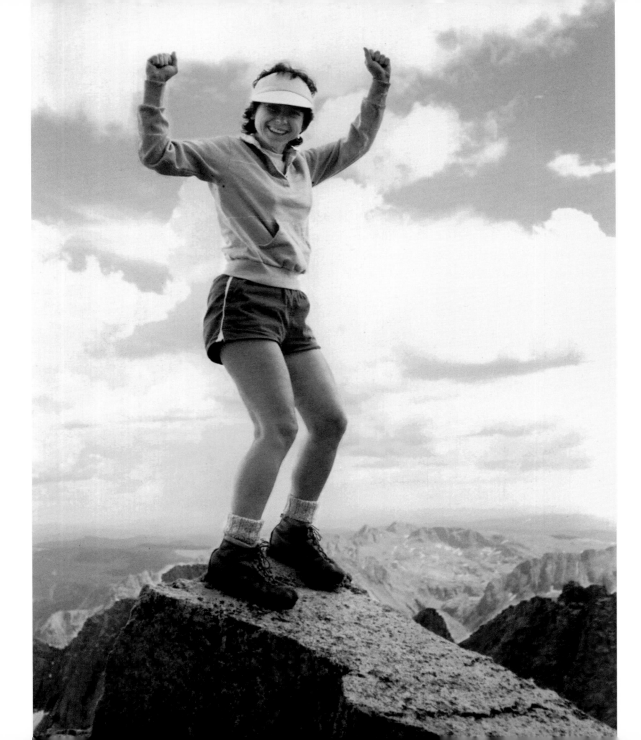

THIS QUIET, MEDITATIVE WOMAN

began climbing her first mountain at the age of 34.

The early hours were filled with great joy and anticipation. Purple, shoulder-high larkspur lined the path and the stream alongside danced in the sun. Soon, however, I rose above the tree line. The air became painfully thin and the path disappeared into a vague impression through treacherous piles of rocks.

I could see the peak in the distance, but I was at the limit of my endurance. My legs ached, my stomach was sick from exertion, my lungs burned.

With one more painful effort of muscles and will, I scrambled to the summit. Mighty mountains spread out around me, below me.

"I am on top of the world," I shouted.

And a new, beautiful woman was born.

Louise
Placitas, New Mexico

I HAVE ALWAYS KNOWN THAT I AM SICILIAN.

Actually, what I have always known is that my grandmother, whom I resemble, came from Sicily. Then one day when I looked in the mirror, I saw it: Sicily. Reflected in the glass was my heritage, my connection to women and men stretching as far back as time. At that moment I was my grandmothers and their grandmothers. All at once my dark eyes and wide hips were sharing the secrets that I had been ignoring all my life. I traced my thick eyebrows and dark mustache and felt the ancient threads that are my ancestors. I touched my heavy breasts and soft round belly and felt the pulse that came from family, my family.

I carry my history in my body and we are beautiful.

Judith
Arlington, Massachusetts

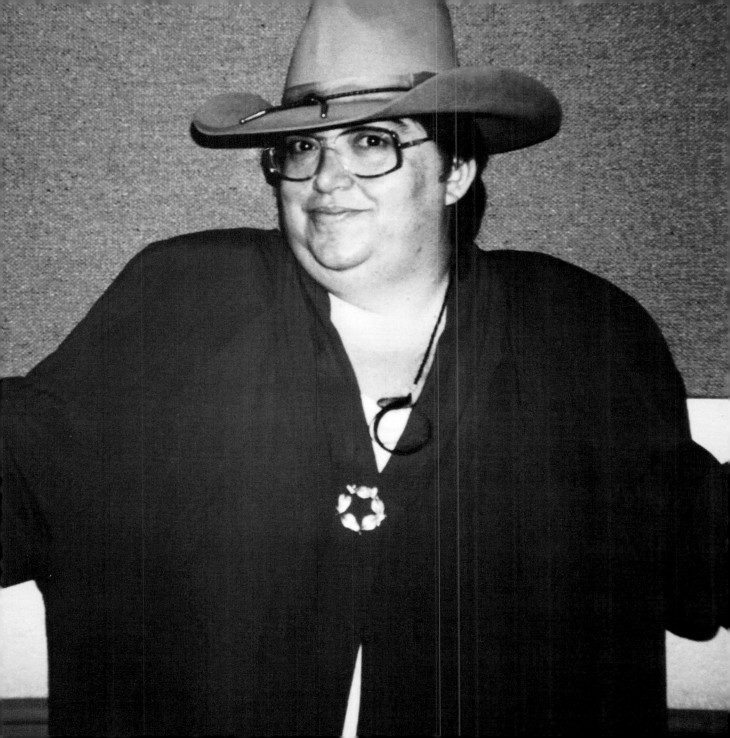

THEY STREAMED INTO MY CLASSROOM,

sunkissed bodies, hair the color of cornsilk or coal, all beautiful co-eds.

Ten years earlier I sat in one of those seats, desperate to learn to write. Now, I was desperate to teach.

"Write," I said. "Write who you are, what you will be."

I expected to read of summer vacations on glistening beaches, goals of TV anchordom, tales of hunks. Instead, I read of external beauty veiling internal anguish: fat, failure, self-doubt, obsessions, alienation from body and soul, fear of their own intelligence and ambition.

For weeks they worked hard, seemingly swept up in the power of their ideas. Yet in their journals, the anguish remained. They looked to me for answers. How could I show them that what we see are shadows of our bodies, refracted by culture? It's not real.

For our last class I stood before them, clutching glossy glamour magazines. "She's somebody else's fantasy," I repeated. Then newspapers: "Here's a woman writhing in lingerie; and men creating world peace. Here's a gal in a towel; and men creating multi-billion dollar conglomerates to create images of gals in towels," I preached.

Weeks later I got a letter from some of my students. Enclosed was the first issue of their magazine: *SmartWomen*.

The inspiration, they wrote, was me.

I've never felt more beautiful.

Pamela with her students
Chicago, Illinois

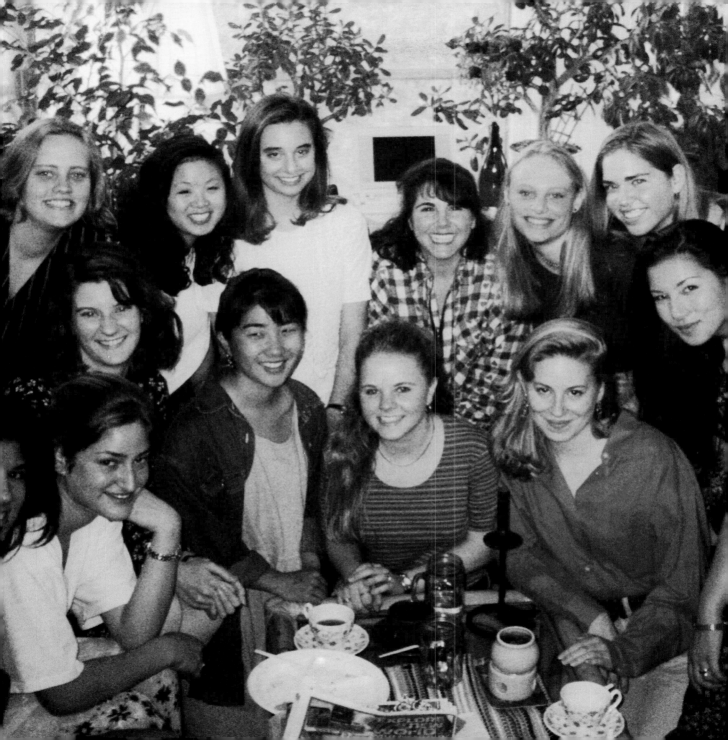

NO ONE HAS ASKED ME WHY

I am beautiful, during my 23 years,
only why I am so strange.
Are they one and the same?
I am a struggling college student aiming for a Ph.D;
I am bisexual;
I wear a backwards baseball cap almost every day;
I am emotionally strong;
My brother is my best friend;
I like to wear black;
I don't chase my cat away when he wakes me for attention at 3:00 am;
I voice my opinion without offending;
Halloween is one of my favorite holidays;
I know how to dream.

And on days I don't believe I am beautiful, I call my mom.

Holly
Oxford, Ohio

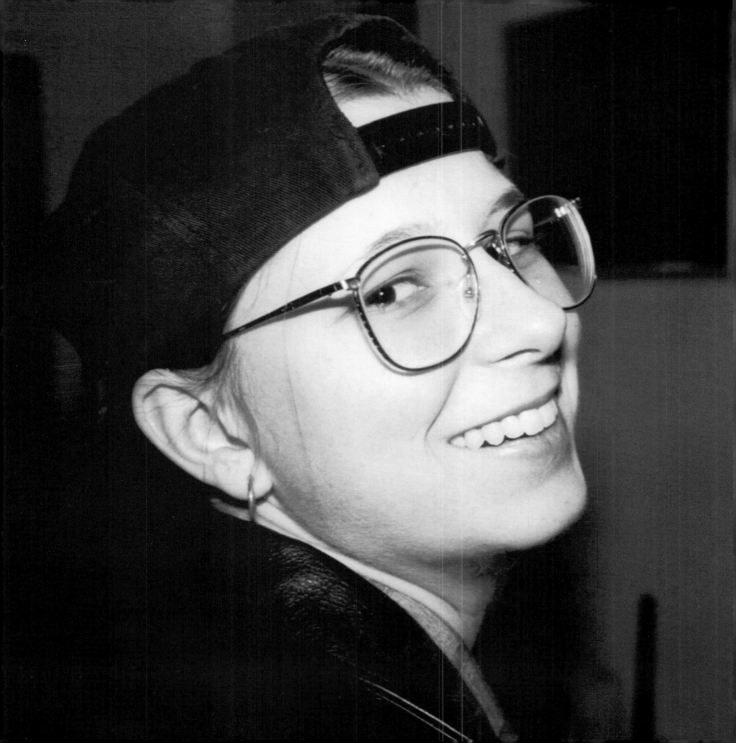

BECAUSE I USE MY HAND TO SHAPE THE LIGHT,

the light that sculpts the image
that reveals what's in my mind,
That shows both bitter loss and blessed grace,
the pushing flesh, the scar you can imagine,
the certainty of death, the hope of life,
I show you the real me,
if incomplete, imperfect,
still struggling, reflecting, and seeking a solution.

Mary
Cranford, New Jersey

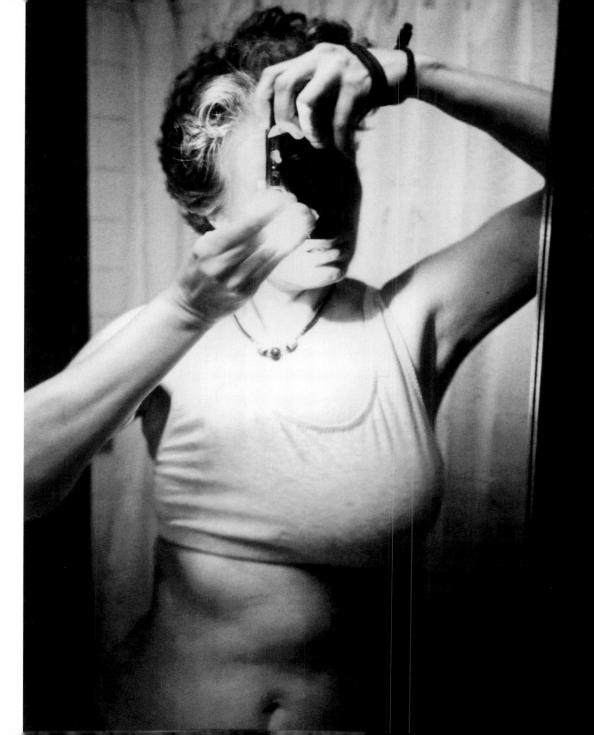

RAISING A FAMILY AND RUNNING A BUSINESS

came before my education. But my desire to learn and to be inspired never rested. So in June of 1994, over 40 years after my original graduation date, I went back to get my high school diploma. Five generations of my family were there to watch me walk across the stage in my cap and gown. Now I am in college.

I have two loving arms, a killer smile, a heartwarming voice, and a listening ear. My heart continues to love with the intensity of one who refuses to know defeat. I continue to live life to its fullest—and that is beautiful.

Lucille
Telferner, Texas

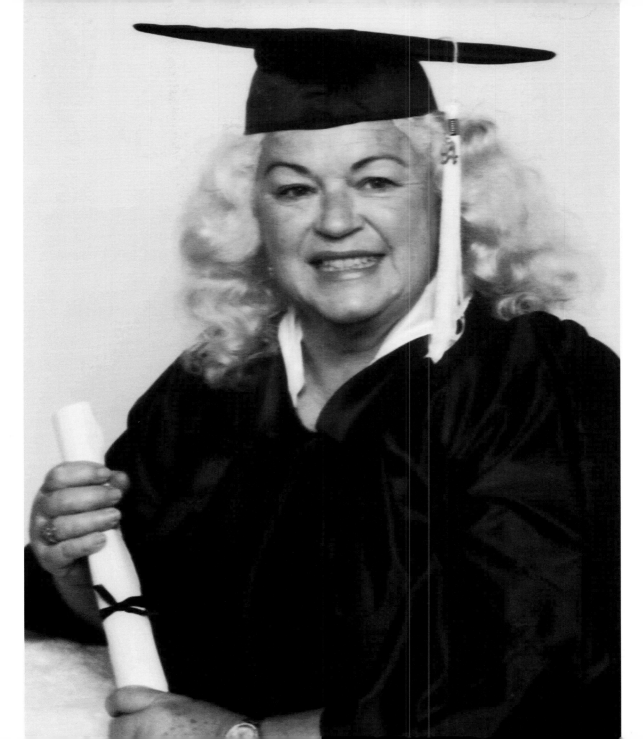

THE BEAUTY INSIDE ME SWIMS UP INTO MOVEMENT,

my dance. It is rarely "pretty"; the honesty and vulnerability of my art is its beauty. It is a river of energy that flows out of my body—hands, eyes, feet, pelvis. This journey of movement streams out into the universe and reflects light and darkness—a shooting star. And it touches others. I give my beauty away.

Peggy
Dallas, Texas

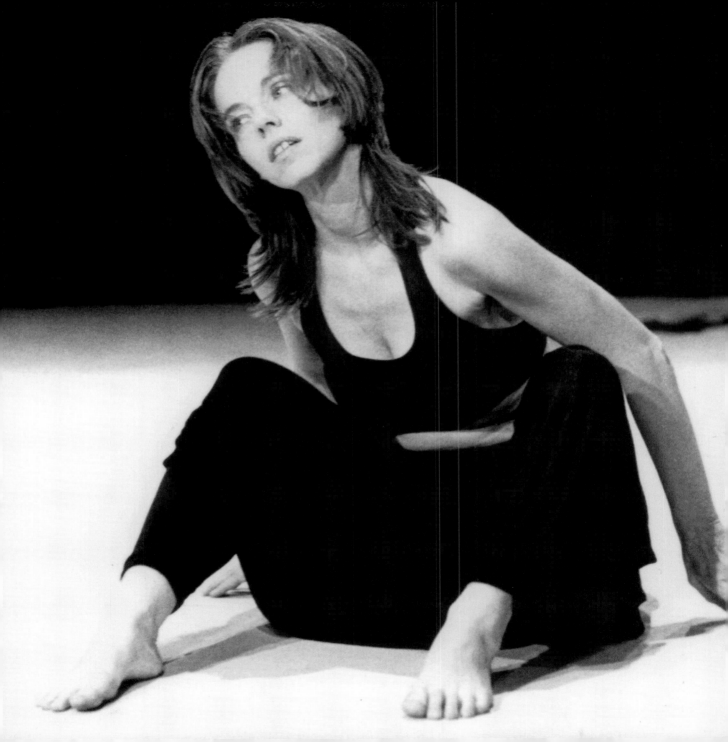

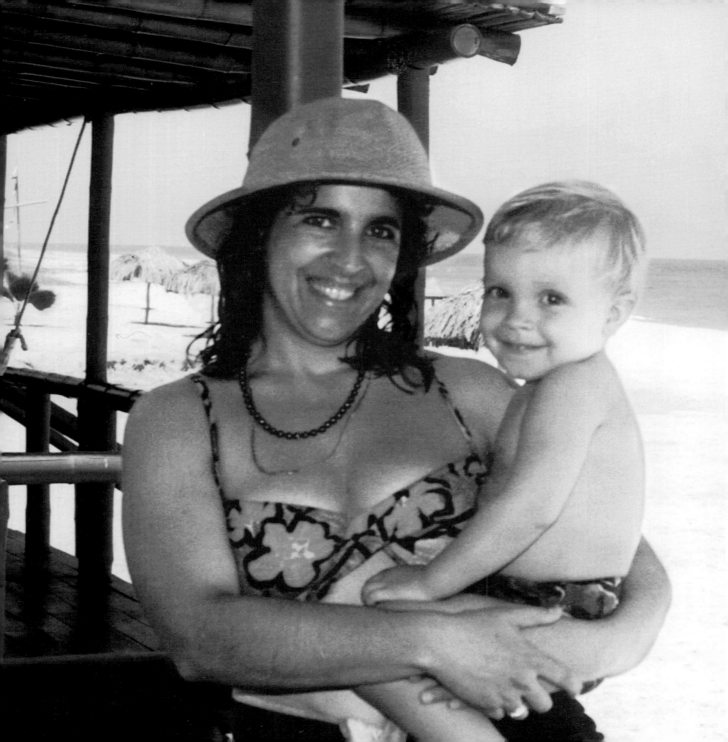

I AM AMAZED

by the most simple and delicate manifestations of life as well as the most exuberant.
I love my planet.
I thrive in human solidarity.
I melt at the innocence of a child.
I am capable of feeling the deepest love in the world. The name of that love is
    Stefan, my sweet son.

And, I like wearing my bikini, even though I'm not skinny. It's wonderful to feel the sun and the water on my belly. Stefan likes blowing in my belly button, too!

Silvana with her son, Stefan
Center Valley, Pennsylvania

I LIVE IN THE PRESENT.

I always try to be learning and laughing. I spend all my money on experiences—airplane tickets, theater tickets, books, and recordings—rather than on things. These experiences, coupled with my pride in my son and the love of my friends, ease day-to-day burdens and transform many problems into challenges.

I am strong. I have survived the deaths of my parents, my brother, my best friend, several cherished cousins, and a marriage. Those and other events in my life have made me strong emotionally. I am strong physically because I swim, dance, and work out.

I am lucky. I do work I love, I know how to spot a whale spout on the horizon, I make the best lasagna you've ever tasted, and I cuddle with my two cats whenever we feel like it.

I know myself, I accept myself, and I love myself. I believe that confidence produces profound inner beauty, which shines right on through.

Patricia
St. Louis, Missouri

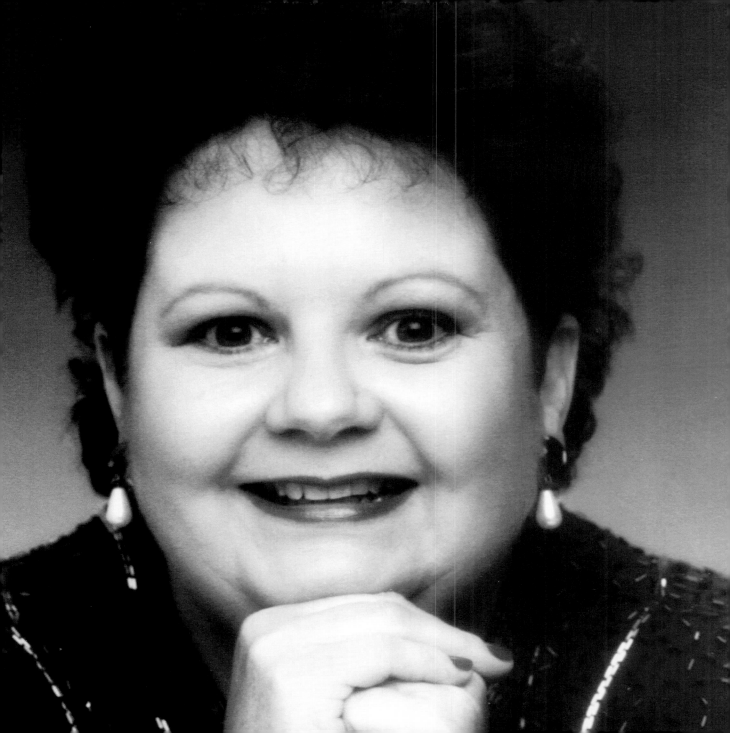

AFRICAN BEAUTIFUL,

full-featured
earth brown
from my wiry, course curls
right down to my well-worn feet.

African beautiful,
worldly wise
analytical and precise,
strong in principles
and culturally aware.

African beautiful,
as softly centered
as the beginning
and as all-encompassing
as time eternal,

a song
and a prayer,
a smile
and a tear,
laughter and curses
all reside
full-bodied, in me.

African beautiful
I know that I am
on every level . . .

But I still need to know
that you know
that I am.

Maaskelah Kimit
Wichita, Kansas

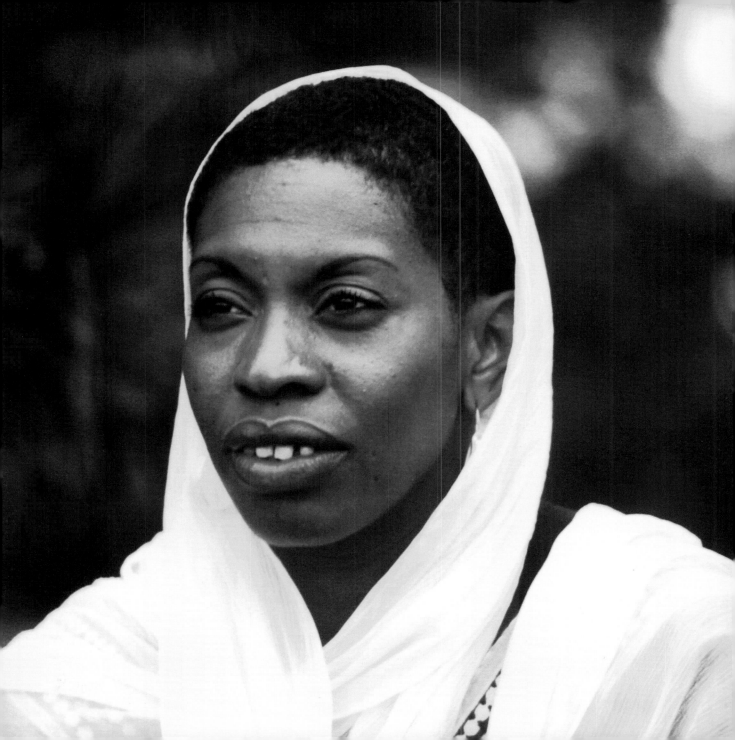

I REALLY DO NOT SEE

my beauty when I look into a mirror; I see it when I look within my soul.

Ami
Fayetteville, North Carolina

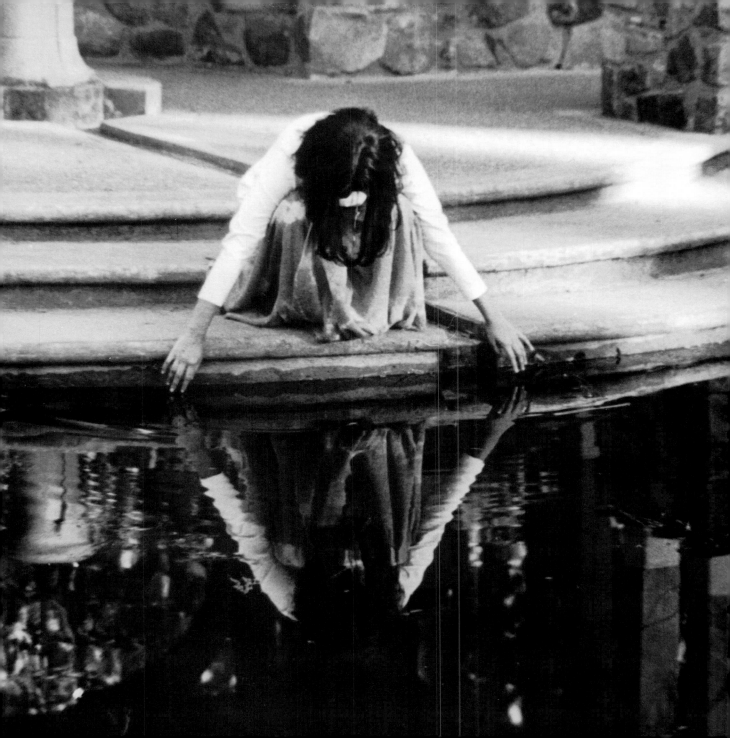

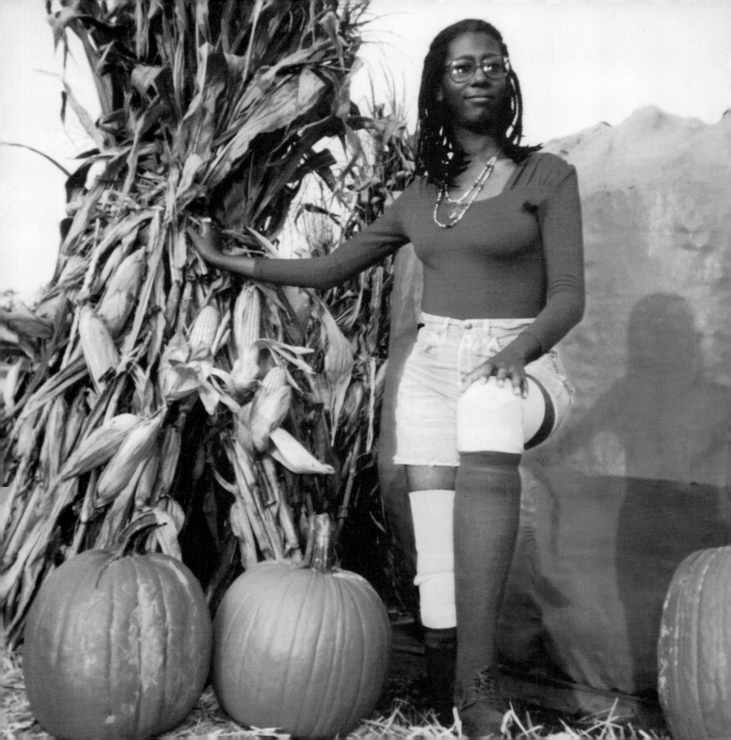

MY TWO LEGS,

amputated below the knees, firmly muscled, carry my lithe body each day on sidewalks, up trees, through crisp air with a sprite-like step, reveling in the peace and beauty of life.

Disabled I am!
    Woman I am!
        Spirit I am!

Shelley
Washington, D.C.

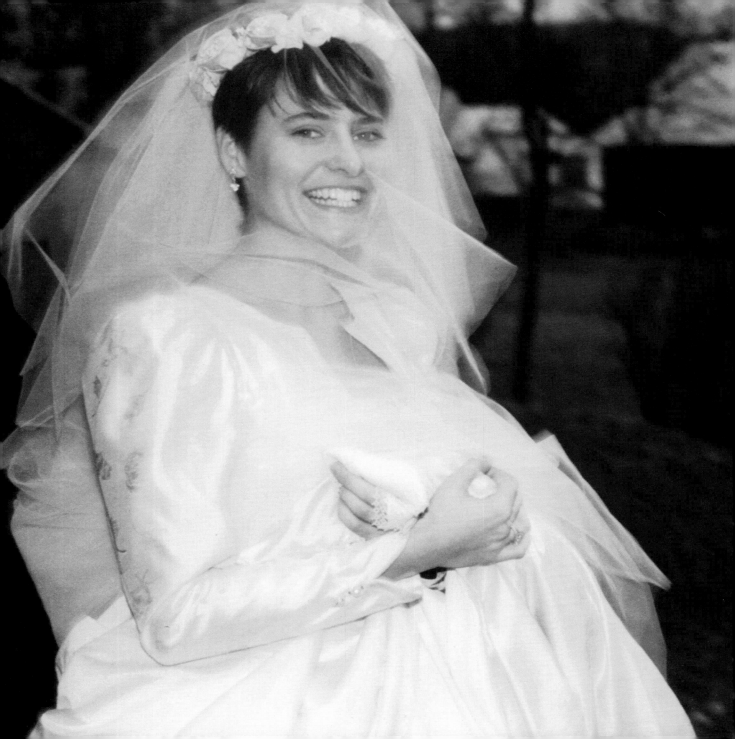

I LOVE TO POP

those warm black tar bubbles on hot country roads.

I gave myself permission to be an artist.

I wore a lovely ivory gown while I walked down the narrow aisle of the little white church, just as my grandmother had 61 years earlier.

I can listen to the wisdom whispered by the voice inside me.

I enjoy a piled-high plate of chicken and biscuits and a blue raspberry sno-cone every August at the County Fair.

I cherish the stretch marks that grace my belly.

I found the person I want to make love to, I want to disagree with, and who I want to play basketball with for the rest of my life.

I let my dog lick my face.

Carla
West Redding, Connecticut

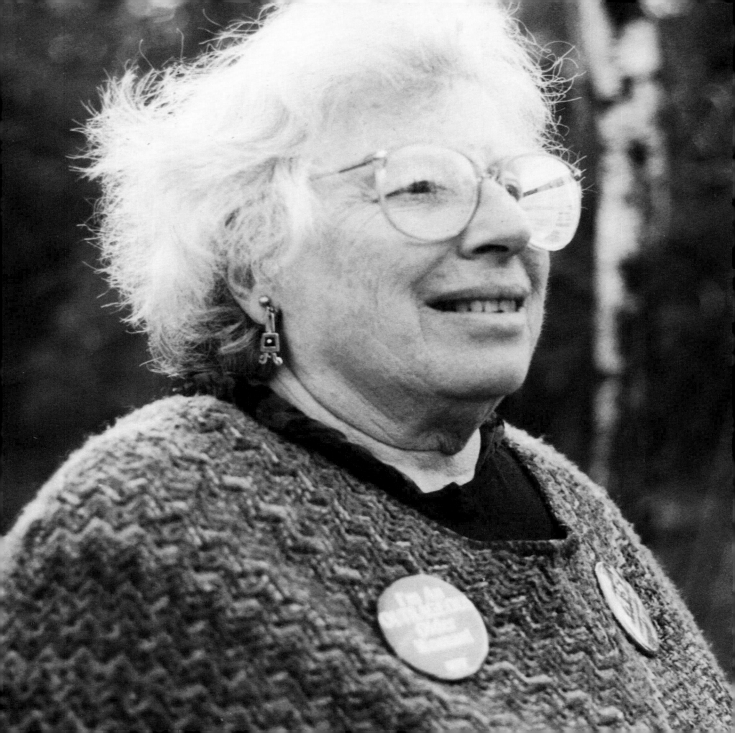

I AM AN OUTRAGEOUS OLDER WOMAN.

Beautiful at age 70 with amazing gray hair and a wonderfully wise face. Truly a late bloomer, I received my B.S. at age 40, and my Ph.D. at 45, and I have authored eight books since the age of 55. I teach and speak around the country. My goal is to share what I have learned with others: to eschew passivity and work to live a life that is full of passion, power, and pride.

Ruth Harriet
Wellesley, Massachusetts

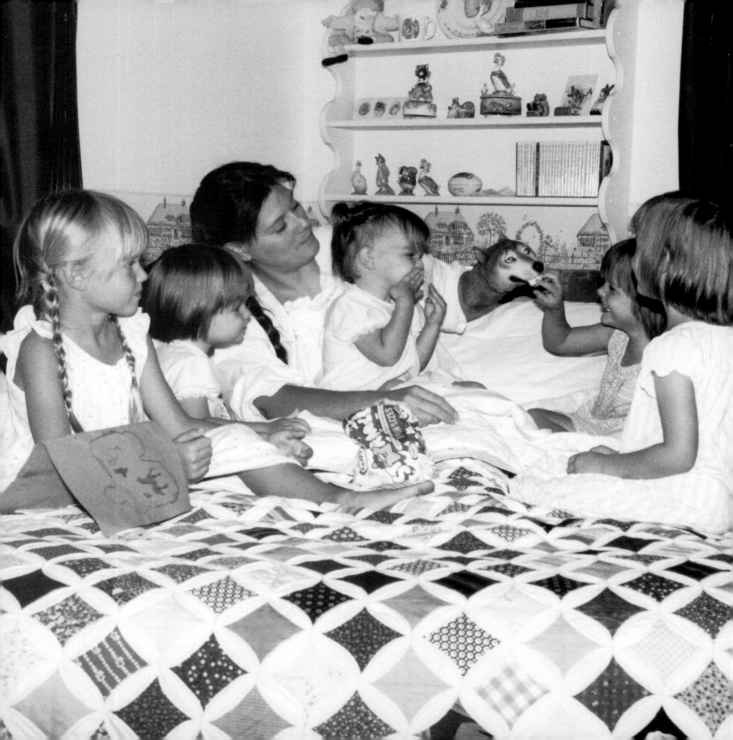

KNEE-DEEP IN DIAPERS,

clothed in the colors of a crayon box, and smelling of freshly bathed puppy, I ask myself: Am I beautiful? The answer is: Every day greets me with five big smiles and five pairs of bright eyes. I know this is heaven on earth. There's no holding back the enthusiasm I have for just living. My little daughters helped me discover there is no limit to the energy I can generate! Painting, drawing, sewing, baking, rolling around on the ground with the dogs, the kids, or all of the above—whatever the activity of the moment, my body will certainly be absorbed in it. Sometimes life makes me laugh so hard I nearly wet my pants.

Jennifer with her daughters, Lucie,
Susannah, Celeste, Lily, and Grace
St. Louis, Missouri

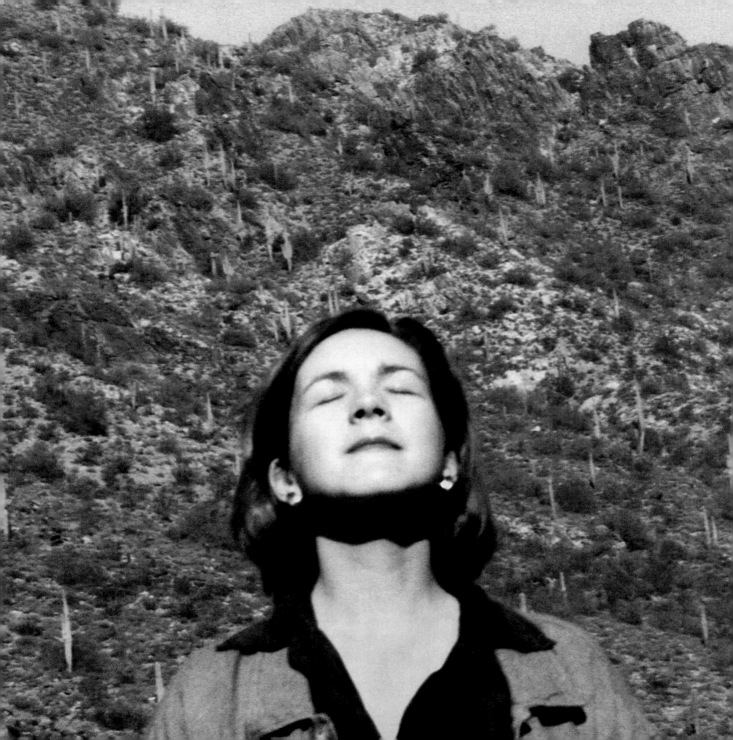

FAR FROM HOME, I AM A WOMAN WALKING THE WORLD —

across great gentle fields, through warm summer seas. I lie on the grass and feel the slight curve of the hill fit to my back. I am a woman lying across the earth. I want to be naked and dancing in the middle of a huge field, arms to the sky and palms open. I create a vision for myself: bold, strong, big, and sure.

I return home, nourished by nature's embrace and sure of her perfection. I take off my clothes and walk onto the patio. I lie full-length on the lawn chair. Naked, I no longer judge my body by how my clothes tell me I should be. With no binding, shaping, hiding, or lifting, this body is perfect. Every curve and soft place is just right. I see myself and today I am beautiful.

Sandy
Phoenix, Arizona

IN THE WOODS,

I no longer sit in judgment of my actions. I rediscover and accept who and what I am. Burdens and despair slide away when I am restored to a natural state of grace. I no longer need to be needed and I forget about self-doubt and perfection. This is where I find the balance between intellect and intuition, reason and emotion, thought and feeling. I renew the vital knowledge that inspires me to create. In that creation, my beauty as a woman is manifested.

Gloria
Walden, Vermont

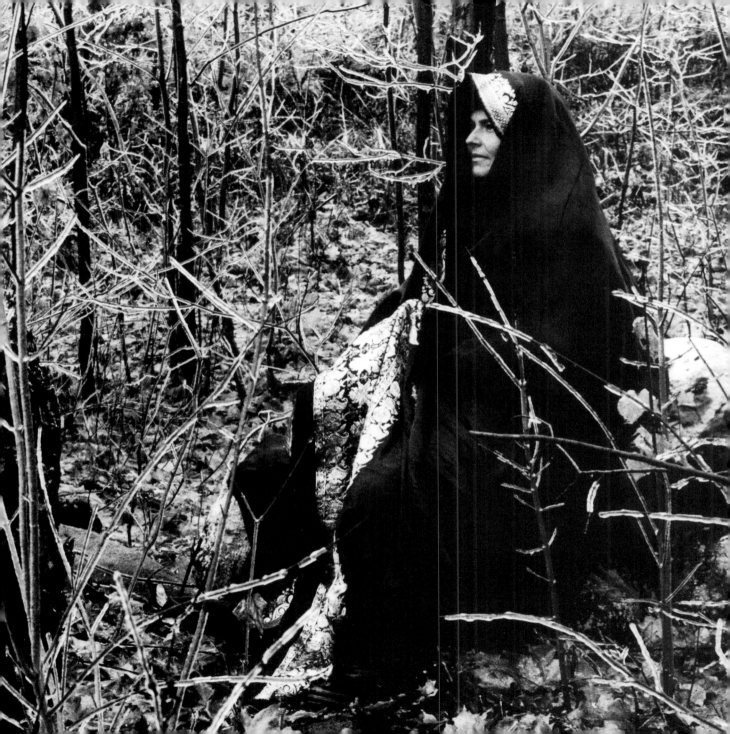

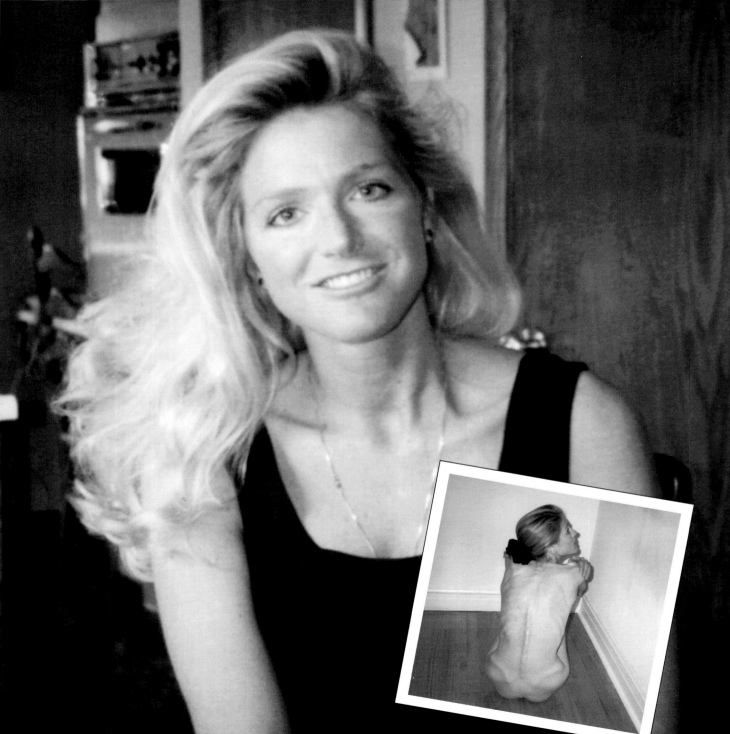

I WAS A LOVELY YOUNG WOMAN.

My soul untarnished by the evils of the world. Not unlike Pandora.

Adolescence unlatched Pandora's box and I became a victim of the dark side of human nature. I was objectified by both men and women. I was stalked like the prey of a wolf. At a tender age I was raped by a man who wanted to have my virginity as his trophy. My innocence, my spirit, my very soul were ripped from me by the crowd that cheered him on.

I punished myself with starvation. It kept me unattractive, safe.
But as in Pandora's box, the final element is hope.

I'm getting back on my feet.
I know I am beautiful inside.
I am beautiful because I am here to tell my story.
I help other women survive rape and find their value in their tattered souls.
I am choosing life over anorexia.
I am beautiful because I am becoming the woman I want to be, the woman I deserve to be.
And slowly, I am learning to smile again.

Carol
Madison, Wisconsin

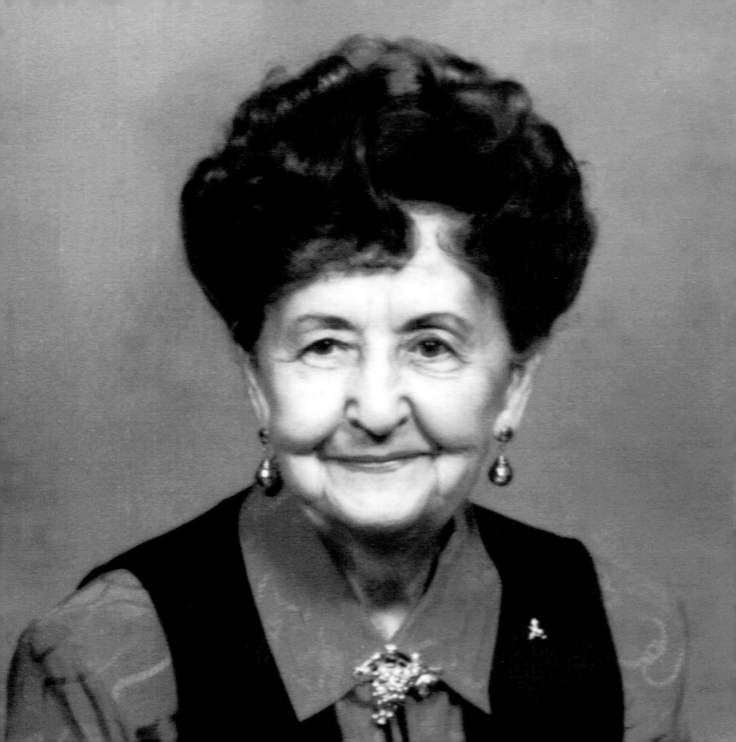

I AM 89 YEARS OLD

and I still drive and participate in all the activities I've ever done. I make someone laugh every day because, to me, humor and laughter are the music of the soul.

Mildred
San Antonio, Texas

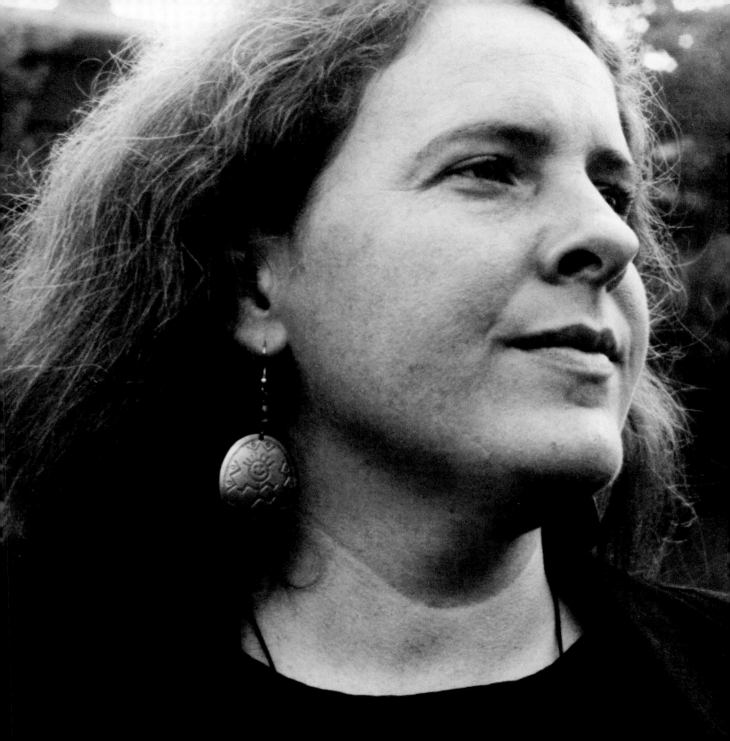

Caught in a Moment between Rushings.

Rushing to the car, rushing children into seat belts, rushing off in the car.
Strength. Calm. Elegance. Seriousness.
I have a sensuous, solid beauty.

Healthy skin, clear eyes, and a strong body grow from my love of cold weather and great food.
Gray in wild, wispy hair shows life touching me.
Open arms signify a heart freely shared.
Sturdy features place me firmly in a line of powerful, salt-of-the-earth women and men.
Lines of thoughtfulness, grief, and laughter tell of a woman who chooses to sit with pain
    until healing brings an easy laughter.

Kathryn Margaret
New Haven, Connecticut

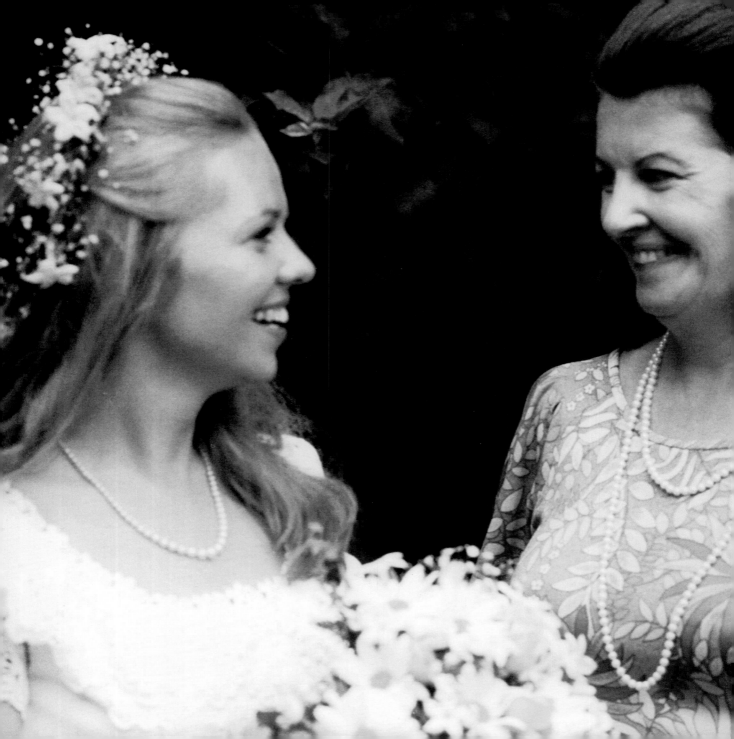

WHEN I LOOKED INTO MY MOTHER'S EYES

moments before my wedding, I felt absolutely beautiful. I could see her joy and pride, and I let her unconditional love soothe my fear of leaving home and living without her.

Fortunately, she continued to be a loving presence for me and my family for 14 years — until she died without warning in her sleep. I never got a chance to say good-bye to her. I've longed to hug her one more time and to tell her how much I love her.

Recently, I noticed how much I look like my mom. Sometimes when I glance in the mirror, I can see her eyes in mine, her smile in mine. Often I can hear her laugh in my laugh. I feel comforted that she is part of me, and I feel more beautiful than ever.

Anne with her mother, Muriel
Oak Brook, Illinois

DISCUSSING MONET'S "WATER LILIES"

with a group of museum visitors, I can open the door to the world of art. When I see a certain look, a smile, or a nod, or hear a question in response to this art, I share the feeling, the excitement of discovery. This is beautiful.

Sari
Clayton, Missouri

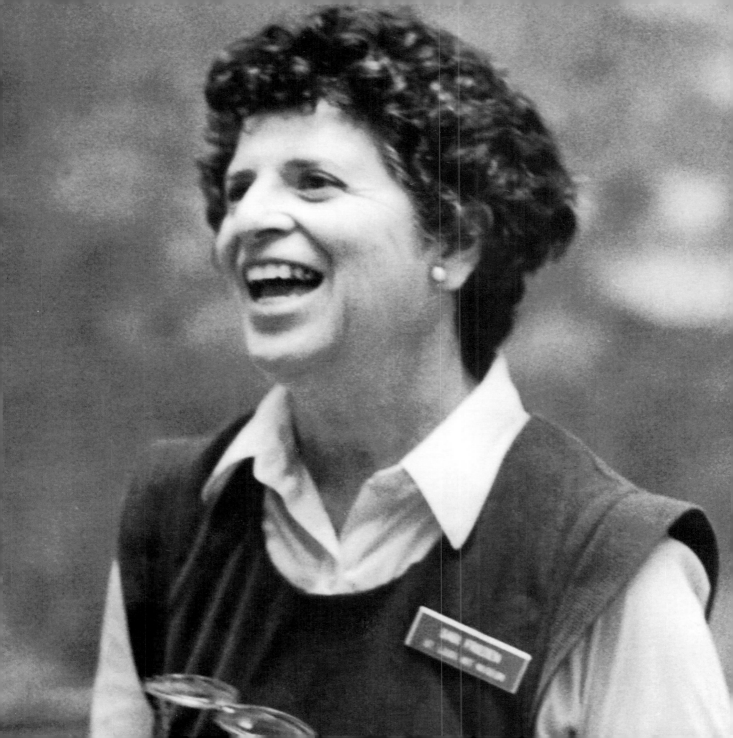

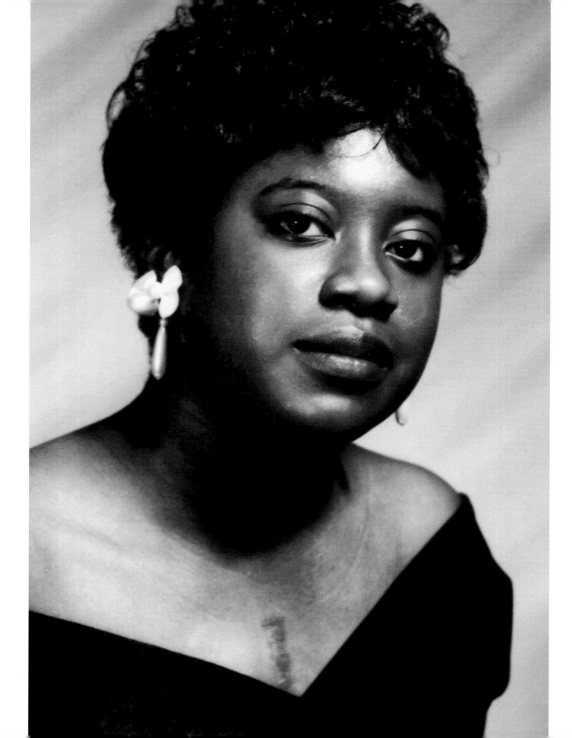

I AM JUST BEGINNING TO FEEL BEAUTIFUL.

Getting past the low self-esteem I had was torture, but I succeeded. I grew up in a dysfunctional atmosphere, was told that I was ugly, faced racial discrimination even from my own because I am not light-skinned or thin with long, weaved hair. A nasty scar from open-heart surgery going down my torso made me feel desperately flawed. Plus now I am fat and have stretch marks from my pregnancy that disgust my son's father.

But I am proud of my scar;
without it I wouldn't be alive.

I am proud of my fat and stretch marks;
without them I wouldn't know the joy of motherhood.

I am black.
I am scarred.
I am strong.
I am proud to say how beautiful I am.

Chanel
Niagara Falls, New York

ONE DAY WE WORE OUR ANIMAL MASKS

into town and shared them with strangers we met along the way. We had a cow scoop ice cream, a hog ride on a Harley in front of a bar, and three boys "sheepishly" fish off a pier. Those boys then followed us through town to see what we'd do next.

Play generates a fountain of youthful energy that removes the wrinkles of time. When you see the world as your playground, opportunities arise. The ordinary begs for a sprinkle of magic. We grab the chance to open a box of crayons and add a mixture of color into the world. As a result, our faces glisten in the afterglow of an afternoon spent romping through life, twinkling with imagination, and swinging on stars.

Kathy and Sue
Whitewater, Wisconsin

WHEN I WAS A CHILD,

my family gave me every opportunity to see myself as beautiful through love, affirmation, and acceptance. I was successful in much that I tried. In spite of that, I wanted to look like the pretty girls and women on the glossy pages of those magazines which brought the definition of beauty from the outside world into my life. This world would someday determine my fate by including or excluding me as student, employee, participant, and partaker. I was at the mercy of a system that would confirm or deny my presence based on unjust rules that I felt could be overridden if only I looked the right way: blue-eyed, blonde, and beautiful.

At age 55 I've learned a thing or two. My discovery that beauty comes from within has taken the place of my need to use others' definitions. I am beautiful because I say I am!

Marian
State College, Pennsylvania

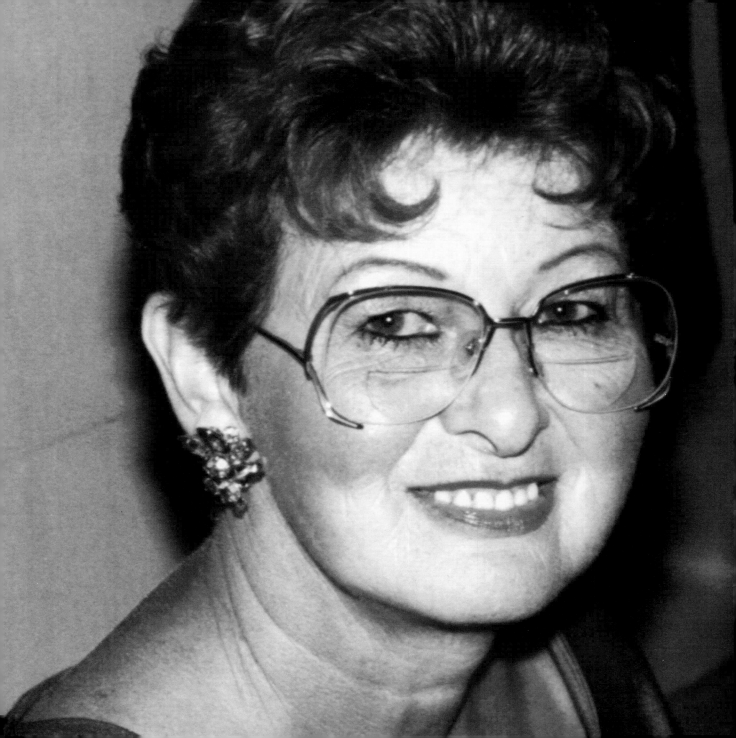

I LEARNED TO ASSESS MY BEAUTY

in the mirror of men's eyes as a young woman in the '50s. Time and time again, I naively sought reassurance of my self-worth in that reflector.

As an older and wiser woman, I have seen every kind of beauty a woman could ever experience. And, ironically, it was reflected in the eyes of men.

In the eyes of my husband, I saw the beauty of true love;
in the eyes of three sons, the magnificence of motherhood;
in the eyes of my grandson, the assurance of the cycles of life.
And in the eyes of young men dying of AIDS, the beauty of a compassionate, loving mother
seen first in the eyes of my son, and then in those of four other mothers' abandoned sons whom
I cared for in my home.

Tess
Houston, Texas

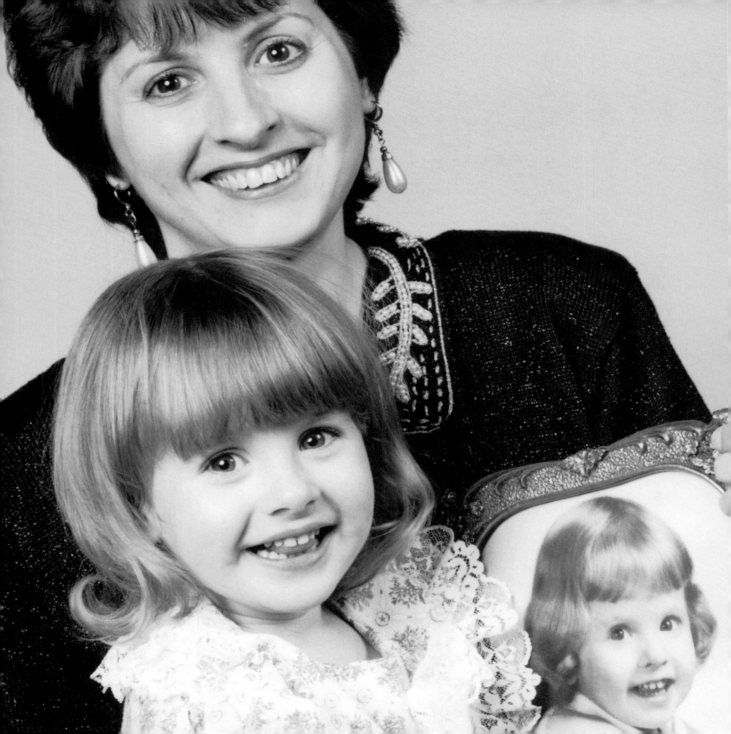

Many times people have told me

that I was pretty or that I looked beautiful, but I never believed them because I didn't see myself as beautiful. Two-and-half years ago I was graced with the gift of a beautiful baby girl. Of course I think my daughter is beautiful—I'm biased, I'm her mom. But I didn't see the remarkable resemblance that almost everyone mentioned.

It was just recently that I looked at the large black-and-white photo of me when I was 18 months old that sits on top of my dresser. It was like seeing it for the first time. The resemblance between me and my daughter was incredible. I kept looking back and forth from the photo to my daughter. I thought how beautiful she is, and then it hit me: I am beautiful too.

I hugged my daughter tight and thanked her for the gift I had just received.

Yvonne with her daughter, Shavonne
Kansas City, Missouri

MY FAMILY BELIEVES BEAUTY IS DENIAL OF THE BODY.

My mother pushed me to eat only in private and to wear black as a way to hide my weight. I lived in a house littered with control-top pantyhose and a refrigerator of food labeled with the calorie count. To lose weight, Aunt Janice ate baby food and vinegar. Aunt Diane drank only coffee while pots brimming with food rotted on her stove. They still see their active denial of need as their strength.

And denial is my strength, too, for I have denied my family's prescription of beauty and stopped this cycle of self-deprecation. I love my body and its uniqueness.

I am beautiful when I am kissing, wearing my new bikini, talking about the forbidden, and eating!

Alissa
Minneapolis, Minnesota

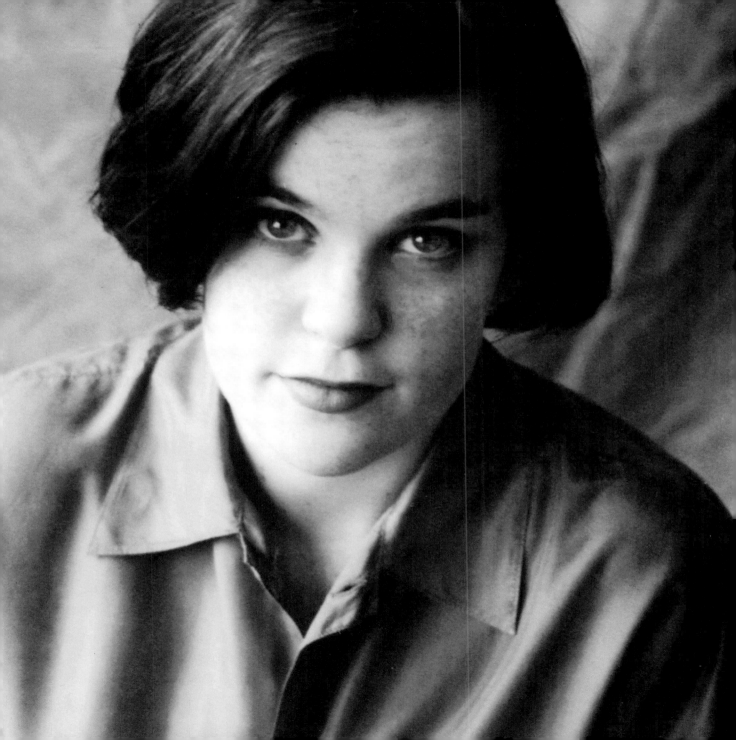

I AM BEAUTIFUL BECAUSE I FEEL BEAUTIFUL.

I move gracefully around the dance floor with steps so intricate that other dancers stop and stare; and I dance every dance with unbounded energy.

I live in the sun, look good in a swimsuit, and my eyes and voice are still fabulous.

Joan with her dancing partner, Phillip
Palm Desert, California

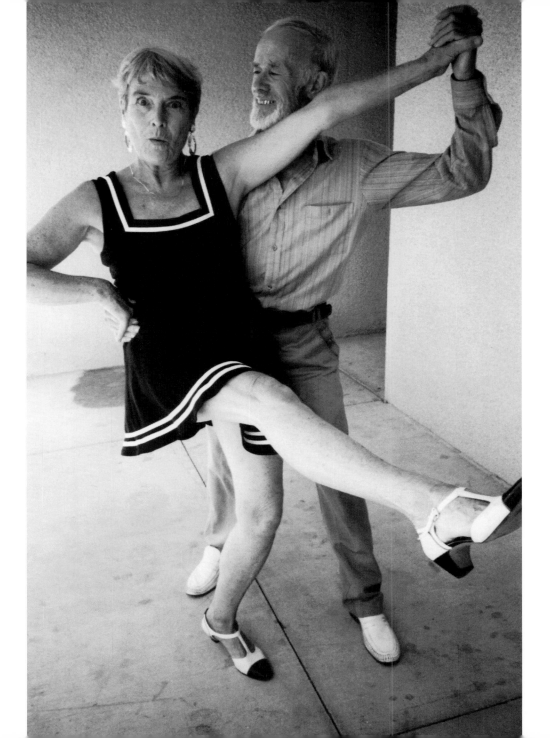

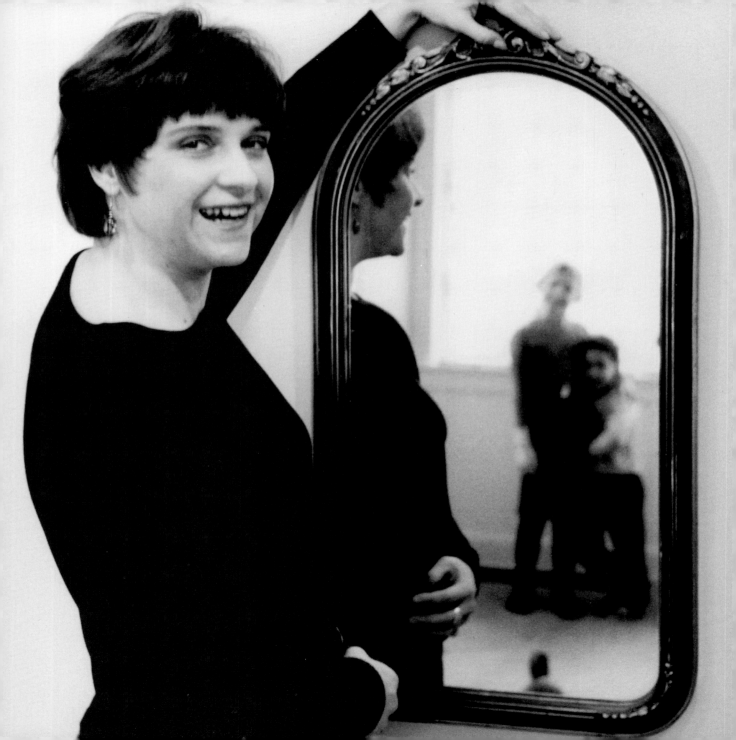

SOMETIMES I LOOK AT MYSELF AND CRY

because I am a 37-year-old single mother filled with grace and passion, and I have no man to witness my beauty. I tell myself that there are other ways to witness the beauty of body and soul, but it's not easy because we are so conditioned to believe that our relationships with men are what define us.

I know that my beauty comes from the joy I find in the simple things—playing with my son, combing my daughter's long red hair, growing flowers, lying in a bed of clean sheets. I cannot deny my desire for a man to witness my beauty, but not having one doesn't make me any less beautiful.

Lynda
Chicago, Illinois

I HAVE SOME GRAY HAIR

and some wrinkles, and I wear glasses, but so what? I still walk tall and straight, feeling the beauty within myself because I am a winner.

My husband and I are cancer survivors. Our experiences have helped give us new perspectives on the world and our role in it. My survival has extended my self-confidence and zest for living. I do feel beautiful inside. Perhaps that shows outside as well.

Margaret
Cleveland, Mississippi

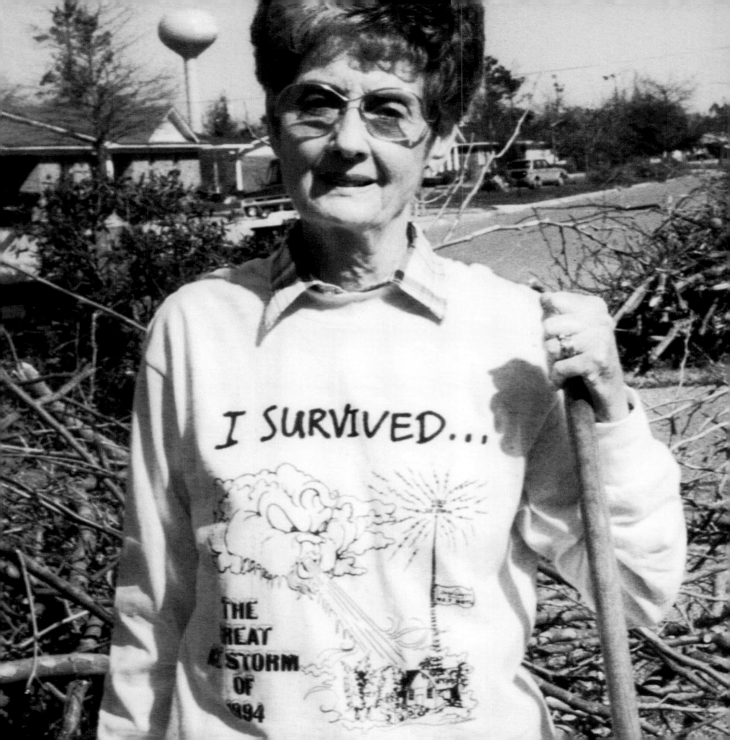

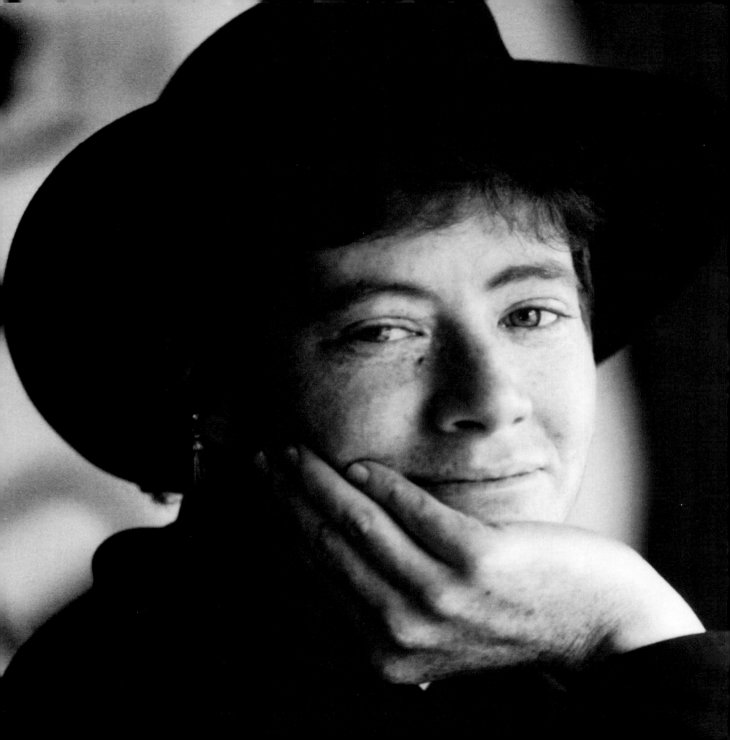

WHEN I LOOK IN THE MIRROR,

I see a fairly attractive butch—one with seductive green eyes, flaming red hair, and an elfin face. These externals don't make me feel beautiful. I know that I am beautiful when I am being creative, singing, writing, and especially, acting. When I draw a roomful of strangers into my world and suspend them in a temporary reality, we click into a single entity, collaborating in an artistic creation. I shine in that connection, and I am beautiful.

Wyrda
Sunny Valley, Oregon

I NEVER FEEL SO WORTHY,

so fulfilled, so humbled, as when I am in the classroom. Each day I confront challenges of every variety, and although I become frustrated and discouraged at times, I am spurred on by the chance to nurture young minds.

This little boy captured my heart and brought out the best in me. He was desperate for every fundamental need of life: love, reassurance, food, and clothing. While my heart broke for him a thousand times, I was also blessed with the chance to lessen the chaos of his existence. I am beautiful in this moment because it is proof that I know, I see, and I feel the reasons to celebrate learning, loving, teaching.

Kris with her students
Edwardsville, Illinois

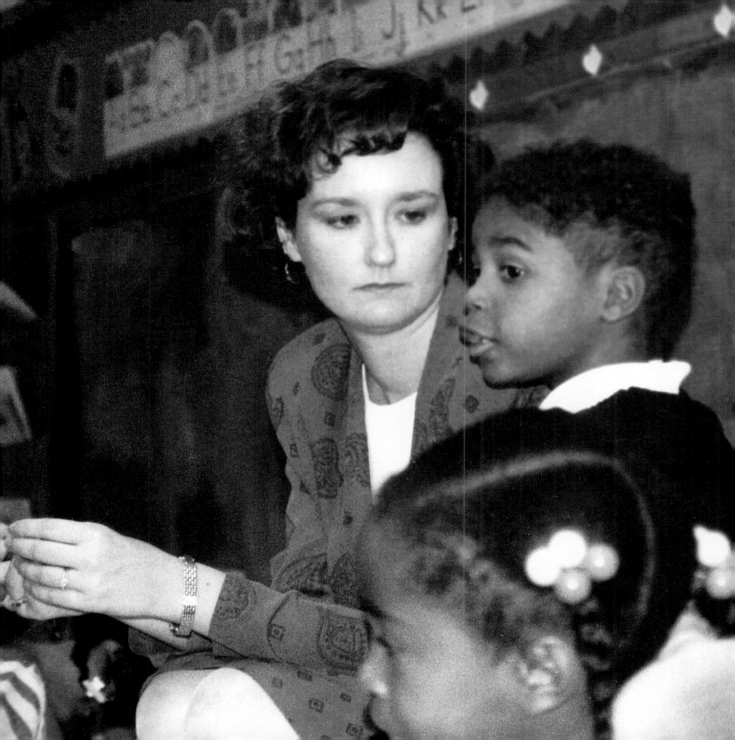

I LOVE THIS PICTURE:

the image and the women are beautiful.
They are as real as any women
real as any
budlightcosmocliniqueladenbathingsuitbeauty
real as any
stickmyfingerdownmythroataftereverytimeieatbeauty
real as any
iwasneverabletolosetheweightafterthethirdbabybeauty.
Real as any woman I've ever seen.

Sarah and Ali
San Diego, California

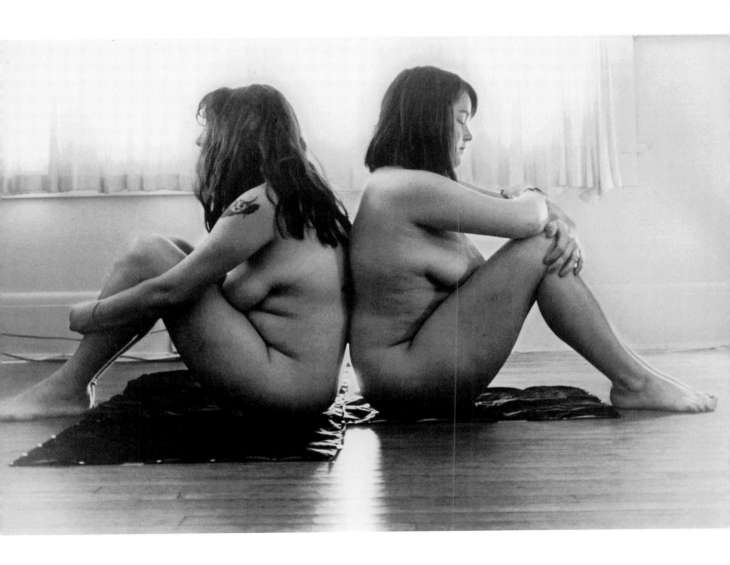

THERE IS A PART OF ME

that remains untouched. It is free from the strain of schedule conflicts, finances, and broken shoelaces. Most of the time I share it with the people I love, but sometimes I keep it to myself and dance.

Catherine
Takoma Park, Maryland

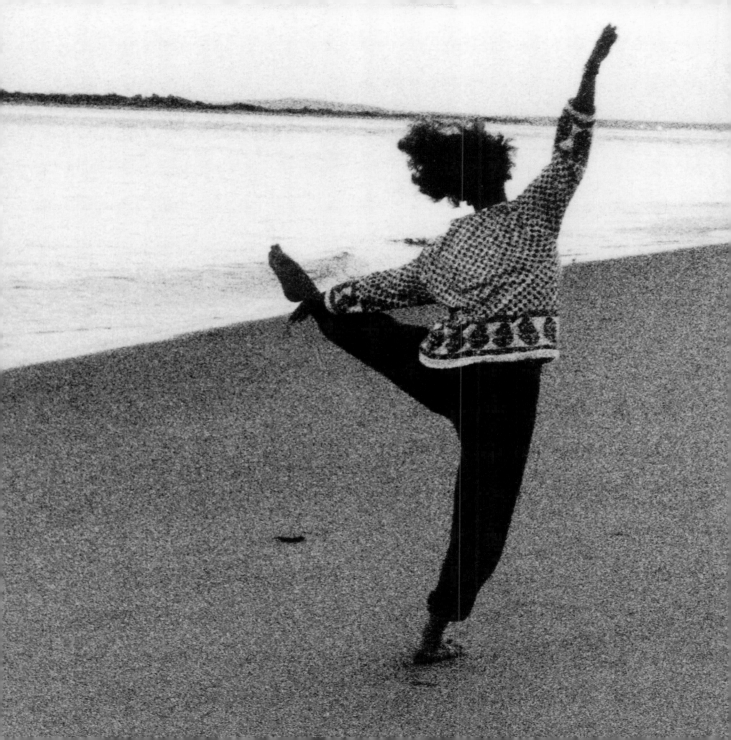

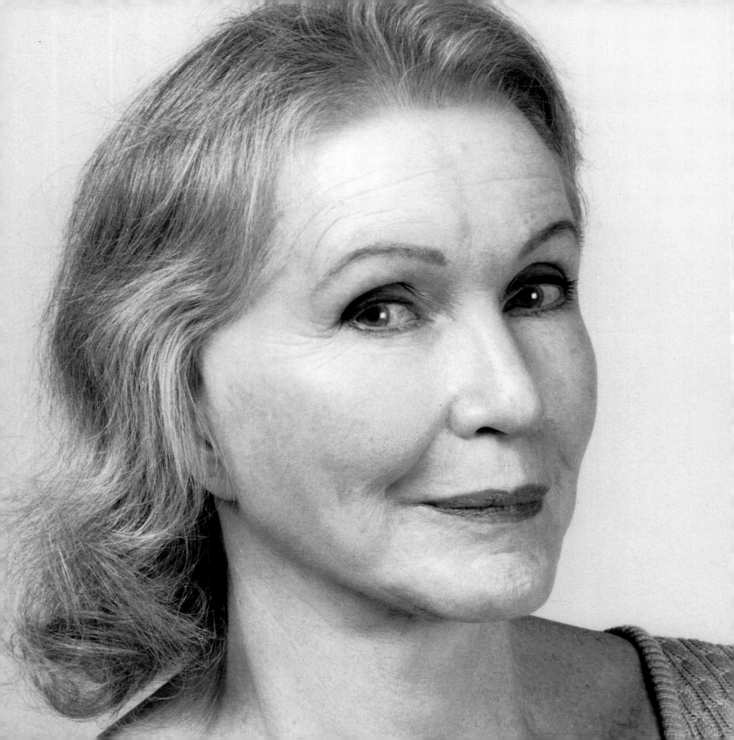

I FOUND MYSELF SOBBING

as I read Clarissa Pinkola's *Women Who Run with the Wolves*. I had spent most of my life unsure of my worth and at the age of 70, I became deeply aware of my value and that of other women. The book tells that within every woman there is a wild and natural creature filled with good instincts, power, a playful spirit, great endurance, and strength, one who is deeply intuitive and fiercely stalwart and brave. Yet, throughout the ages she has been demeaned and harassed, her natural cycles forced into unnatural rhythms to please others.

I like to think that in my 72nd year I have a grace that took all my life's experiences to foster. The humiliations, the hurts, the triumphs, and the loves are written on my face. I was always a woman who ran with wolves. I just didn't know it.

Muriel
Freedom, California

I AM 46,

by far the oldest mother of any first grader in my son's class.

And, this is how I think I am most beautiful: Here I am, looking with perfect love at this little miracle who was born to me when I was 39 after a very high-risk pregnancy. I lost my first child at age 20, and it took me almost 20 years to find the courage to try again.

And now, as this picture reflects, I share the tremendous love and joy we have for each other.

Miranda with her son, Brian
Shorewood, Wisconsin

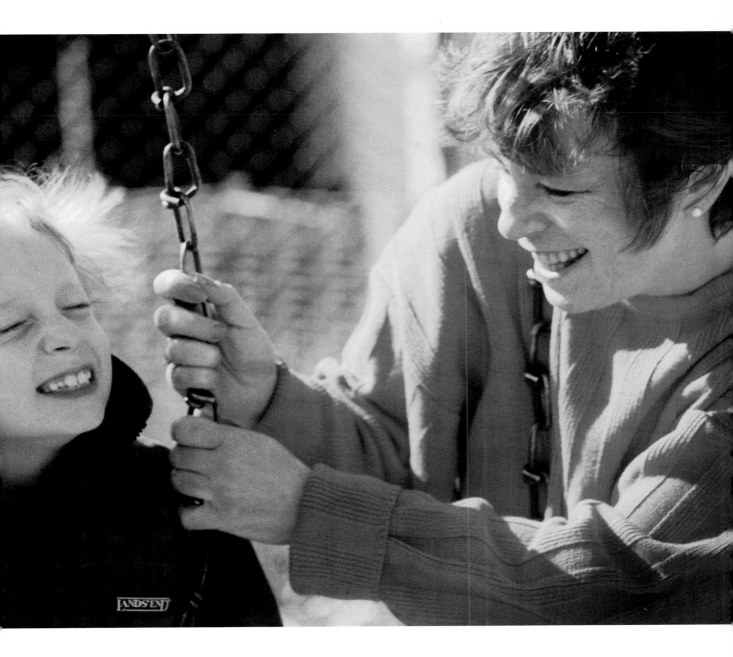

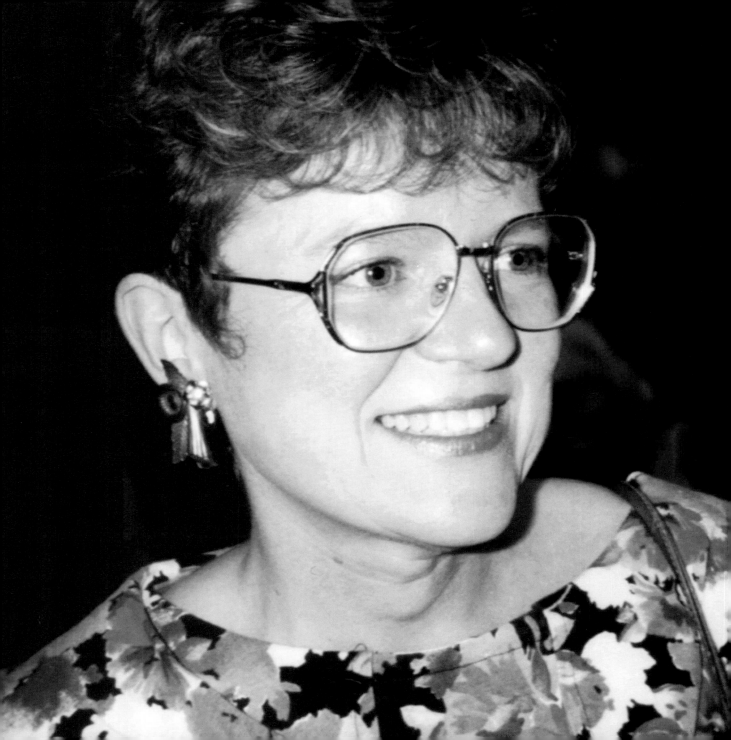

FOR YEARS I BELIEVED THE MEDIA MYTHS

about what a modern woman should be, and forced myself into an ill-fitting mold in an attempt to do it all. I denied my creativity and nurturing side, and simply went through the motions of working to bring in extra money for my family. After a life-threatening bout of depression, I did some reappraising.

With the complete support of my family, I quit my office job and began to focus on what I really wanted and needed to do. I dedicated myself to the full-time spiritual, emotional, intellectual, physical, and creative nurturing of my family—including me! I also began to discover my gift for writing, which I had allowed to lie dormant.

The results of the changes I made have been miraculous. Today I am strong, healthy, balanced, and dare I say it? Yes, I am beautiful.

Cindy
Murfreesboro, Tennessee

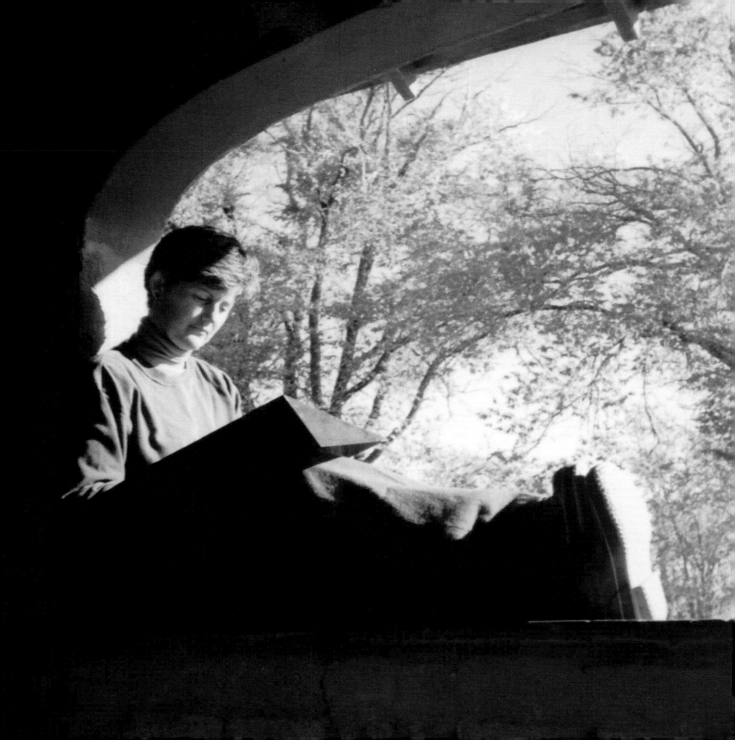

I AM 40, GRAYING FAST,

getting a belly and wider hips. When I was young I swore this wouldn't happen, and I even mapped out my goal weights until age 80 or so. All that changed recently when a 100-year-old woman from the nursing home where I work whispered into my ear, "Watch what you eat, girly. Why, look at all those other women's butts. Don't you ever look like that. That's why I only want milk at lunch, so I don't get a big butt like the rest." With that advice, I decided I really don't want to be worrying about my size at 100.

I've been searching on a deeper level to discover my beauty. I started by returning to school to dispel my old belief that I'm stupid. In developing my mind, I've discovered that I have one. I've also found out that I have needs, I have a voice, I am beautiful. And I have the rest of my life to figure out what I want to be when I grow up.

Rahven
Fort Collins, Colorado

THE MORE I LIVE, THE MORE I LOVE MY BODY.

My legs that have walked thousands of miles on this Earth.
My powerful arms and delicate hands with female fingers and
rings of silver and gold on them.
The curve of my hips,
the muscles of my buttocks.
The dolphin-tattoo on my belly.
My plump lips,
blue eyes,
and pointed ears.

I love it for its beauty and strength.

Tatyana
New York , New York

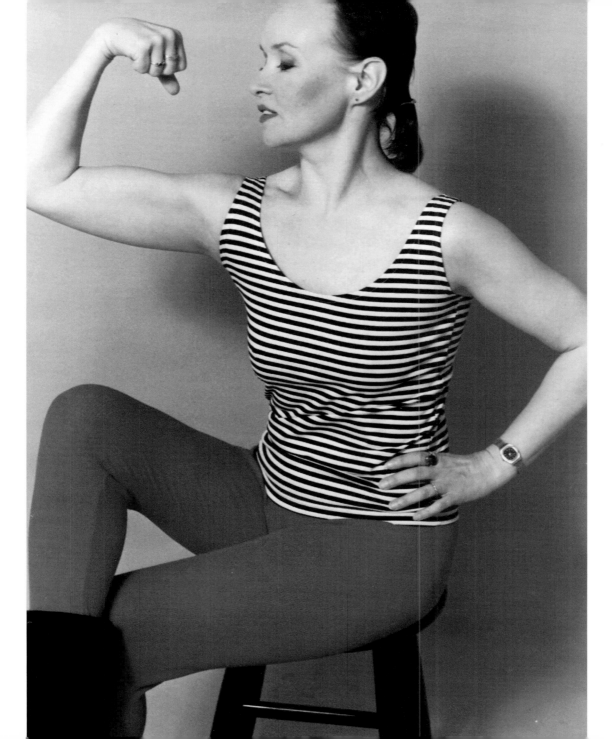

ONE UNSHOWERED AND UNSHAVEN MORNING

I thought, if beauty is not what is outside of me it must be something from within. I quickly disrobed, turned on some music, let my feminine beauty loose, and captured a moment that transcends its time. Beauty is honesty. It is about being real and true to yourself. It's a purity of heart that is uncontaminated by social forces. It's introspective. It's loving and trusting yourself. It's intuitive. It's naked. It's in my tears and in my smiles, and it's mine.

Jill
Boca Raton, Florida

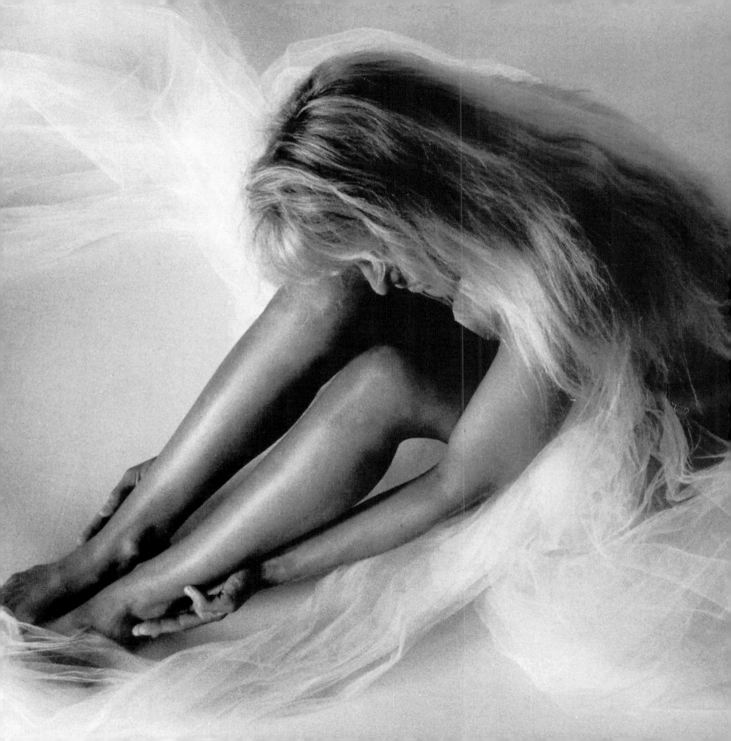

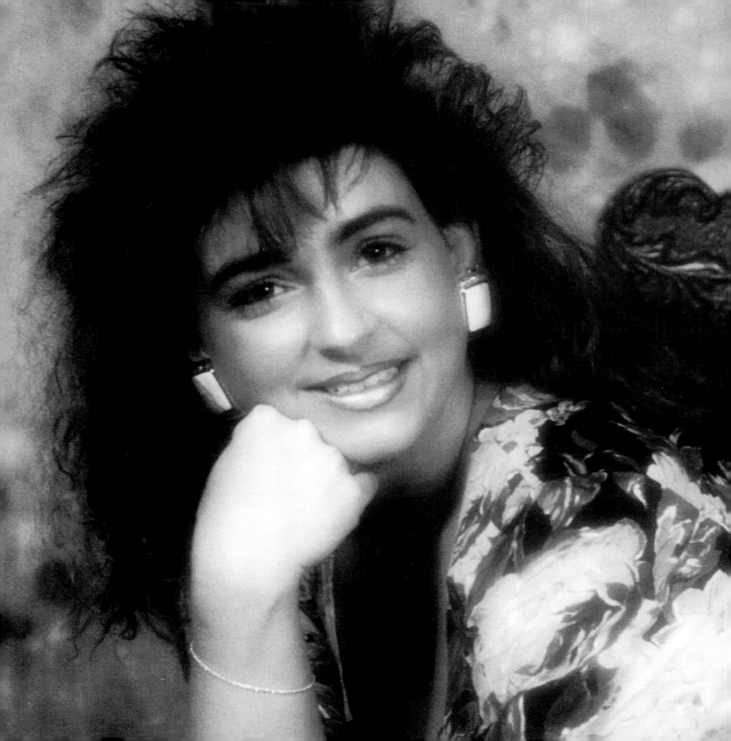

Iᴛ ʜɪᴛ ᴍᴇ ᴏɴᴇ ᴅᴀʏ

as I was brushing my freshly done acrylic nails through my hair, being careful not to snag them on my new weaved-in hairpiece, that all I do to try to be beautiful really isn't what makes me beautiful at all. I thought about having used a straight pin to separate my eyelashes after applying six coats of mascara. I had risked blindness in order to have thick lashes. This is truly sick.

My true beauty comes from my heart, my mind, my very soul. Having survived sexual abuse, having a baby at age 14, working to put myself through college, having my second child at age 23 while in an abusive marriage, divorce, the death of my ex-husband, and the death of my boyfriend six weeks later, my beauty must exceed all stereotypes.

I am strong and smart. I am courageous, generous, empathetic, sensitive, and funny. I can acknowledge that I am really something. And I thank God for letting me see past the lines and the bad-hair days to see how beautiful I am.

Katrina
Nicholasville, Kentucky

To students, a teacher's outer beauty is insignificant.

The inner beauty—how do you treat me, can you help me discover something about the world, do you care about me?—that's all that matters.

When a student discovers the power of his written word
when she sees her writing in print
when he creates a poem that uncovers a truth about life
when a work of literature moves someone's soul
when a class suddenly laughs out loud at some unexpected comment
when a student opens her heart . . .
I am there and I am beautiful.

Vicky with one of her students
Lombard, Illinois

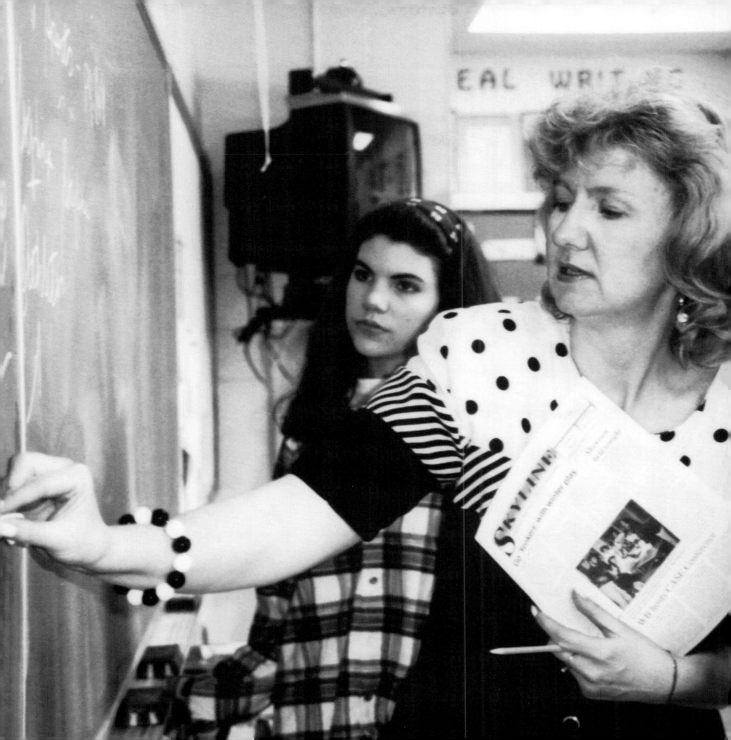

EVERY MORNING AS I AWAKE

beauty begins to flow abundantly about me.

The smell of bacon frying in the cast iron skillet, black and beautiful just like me.
Morning hugs from the children, black and beautiful just like me.
A kiss from my strong, handsome husband, black and beautiful just like me.

Every night as I go to sleep, I notice the evening quiet set aside by God for a special purpose, black and beautiful just like me.

Clarice
Mountlake Terrace, Washington

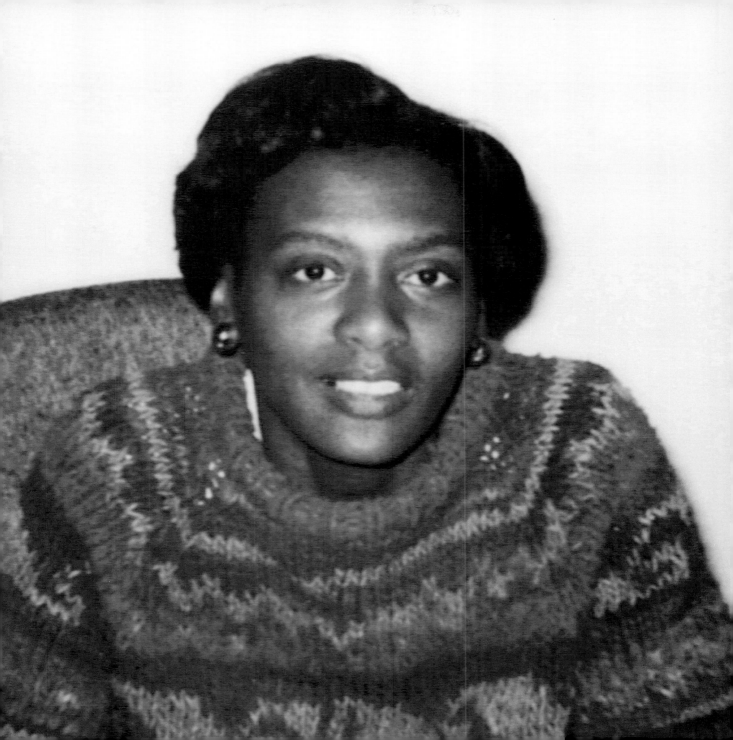

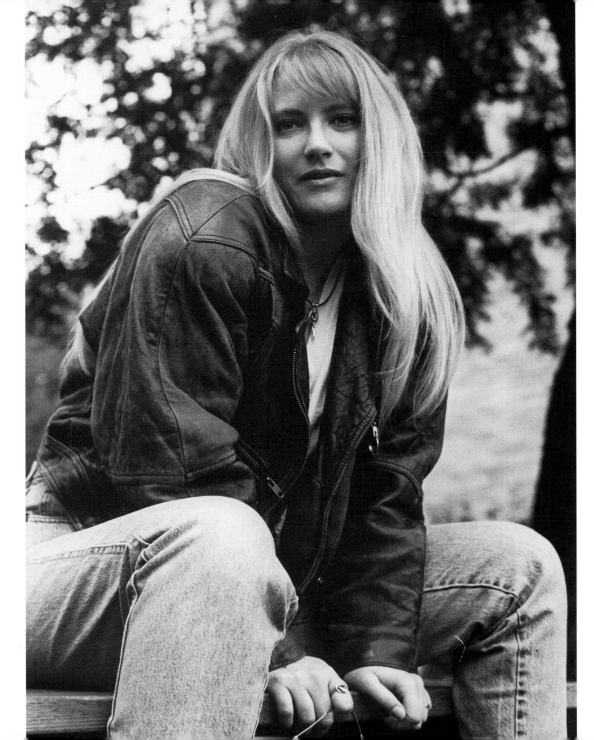

MY FATHER TAUGHT ME

beauty lies in inner strength. My mother died when I was quite young; as a single parent my father has always shown me compassion and discipline, strength, and intelligence. He is the strongest person I have ever known.

I have gained a true appreciation for the environment from my father, the great nature lover. He was always so patient during my early years of temper tantrums and preference for sitting home talking on the phone over cross-country skiing with him in the freshly fallen snow. Not too long ago, I was sitting in the woods with him, feeding birds from our hands, when all that he taught me clicked for me.

In that moment I knew the beauty of my own strength, and the gift my dad has given me.

Elizabeth
Oshkosh, Wisconsin

THE SMILE YOU SEE ON MY FACE

comes from the beauty of my family. My husband, two children, grandchildren, and great-grandchildren are my life. Their love for me makes me glow.

I thank God every day for this beauty. When you have this much love you can't help but feel beautiful.

**Mary with her grandchilden,
Brandon and Ashley**
East Leroy, Michigan

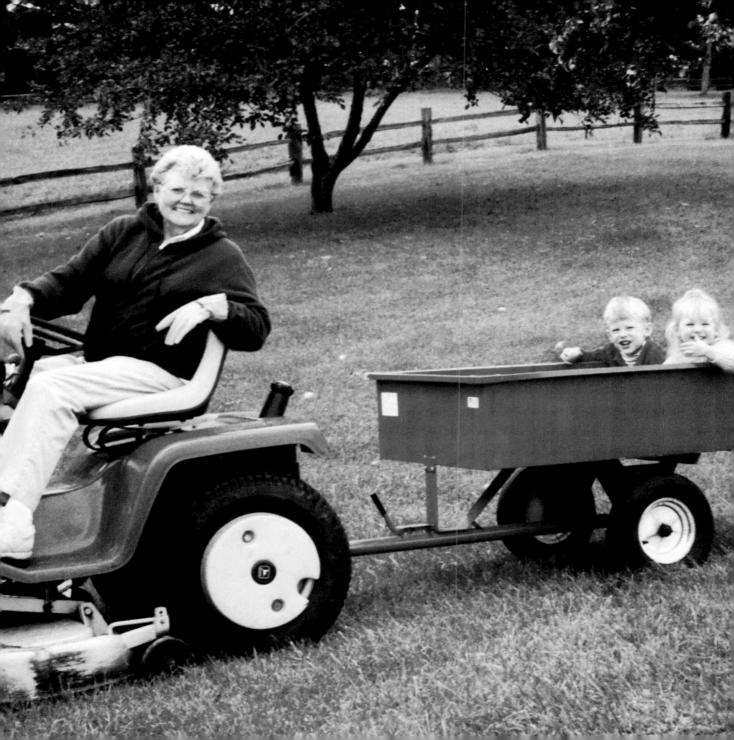

"IT'S NEVER TOO LATE TO HAVE A HAPPY CHILDHOOD."

Words on a t-shirt that turned my life around.

My mother died when I was 3, leaving my father to take care of eight children. He gave me to an aunt and uncle with whom I moved away. One of the first places I remember my aunt taking me to was an orphanage. She explained all of its horrors and concluded our visit with these words: "If you ever get in my way or do anything that I don't like, this is where I will send you."

When teachers inquired about my bumps and bruises, when my doctor tried to get me to tell how my nose was broken, when hospital workers would wonder aloud about how I could be so clumsy, when family friends asked why I was so withdrawn, I remembered the orphanage and I kept silent.

Finally when I was 10 and my aunt was hitting me, I backed her into a corner with a butcher knife. I told her that if she ever hit me again I would kill her. Like the 3-year-old believing the orphanage threat, she believed me. We lived in silent hostility until I left at age 18.

I sought help. I got married and had three sons. I sang, worked and played, but always the happy child eluded me. And then, I found the t-shirt in a gift store, and I knew what to do.

I went home and put up pictures of the sad, hurt, angry child in my bedroom and talked to her. Over and over, I assured her it was not too late to be happy. And I set about making it so.

This picture of me at age 50 shows the happy childhood I am in the process of finding everyday. It was taken at a St. Louis Cardinals ballgame where the child is free to yell, cheer, boo, and generally revel in the gift of life.

Peg
St. Louis, Missouri

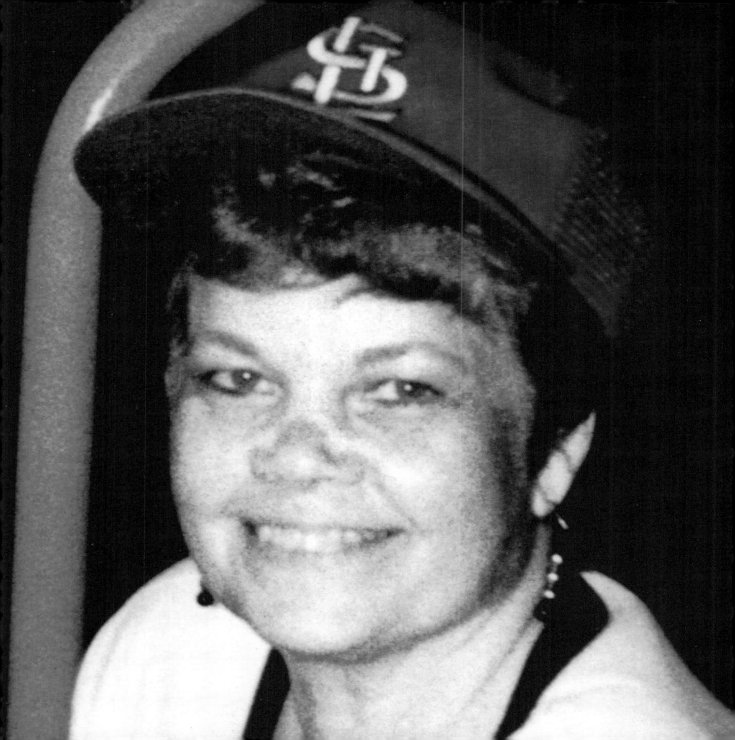

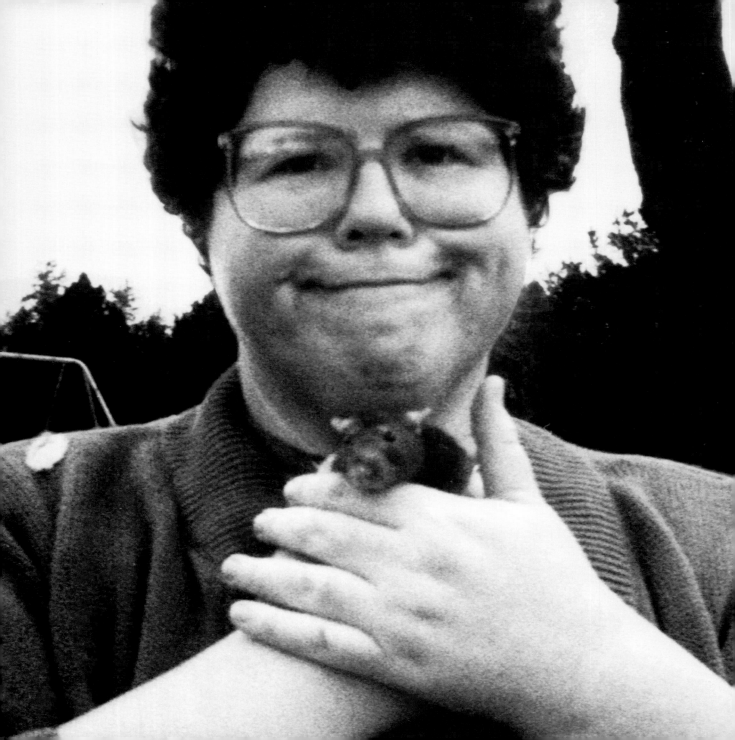

I CAN HOLD A RAT

And make a funny face
Just to induce a giggle from a child
As she snaps my picture on a playground.
That's beautiful.

Julie
Santa Cruz, California

I CELEBRATE MY UNIQUE GODDESS BODY.

I honor her sensuality, her sexiness, her erotic being, her blood, her flesh, her fire, her core of womanness. The large, ample woman's image is the creative inspiration for my work in porcelain and for my spirituality. I do the Goddess' work on Earth in this body that reflects her power, strength, and endurance.

Patrikyia-Sophia
Camden, Maine

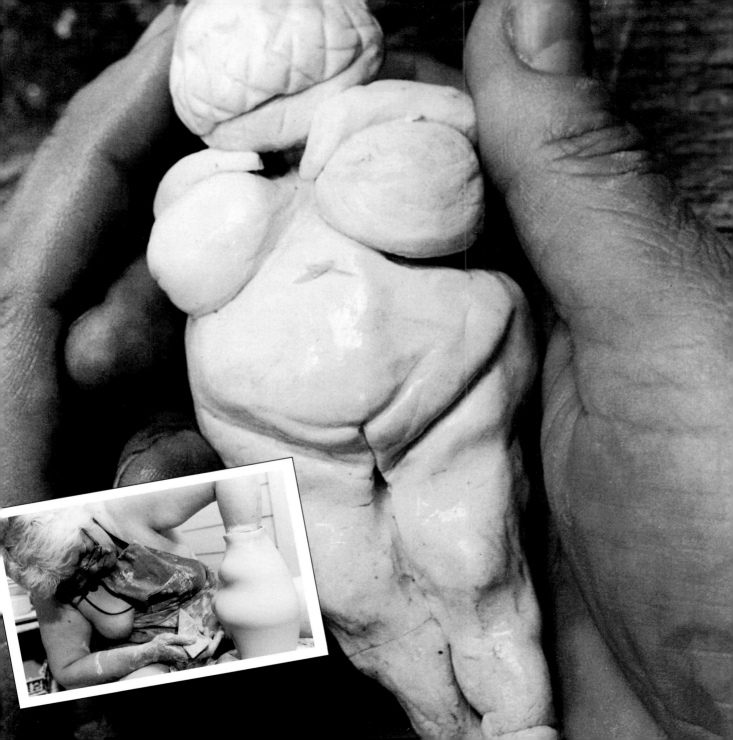

WE'RE BEAUTIFUL BECAUSE WE ARE FAITHFUL.

We've been best friends since kindergarten.
We have run the gamut of emotions: from jealousy to joy; from anxiety to adoration.
We know each other better than we will ever know our husbands. There is a bond that won't break—it won't even crack.

We write, we don't write. We call, we don't call. We live thousands of miles apart, but we always, always know what is going on in each other's heart and homeland.

We're beautiful because we are growing old so gracefully that neither of us can see the fine aging lines and lumps.

Although our surfaces are very different, we share one heart—one side is silver, the other gold.

Sally and Linda
Kentfield, California and Long Beach, Indiana

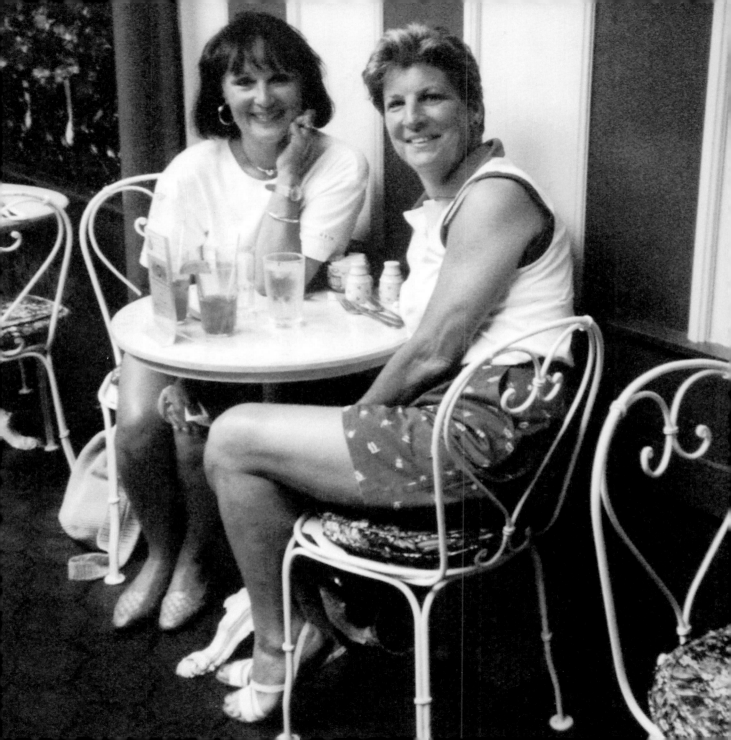

MY BEAUTY BEGINS WITH MY FAMILY.

My father has given me stories, beautiful works of art that he created, and best of all, my nose. My mother has bestowed on me her sense of adventure, her strength, and her passion for films. My sister's charm and wit put a song in my heart.

In sharing the pleasures of sound, sight, smell, taste, and touch with my friends, I feel beautiful. Some friends live only in memory, some are a pounding thunder in my heart. With them, I find my true self.

The love of my friends and family has the power to make me feel like the most beautiful person in the world.

Jen
Washington, D.C.

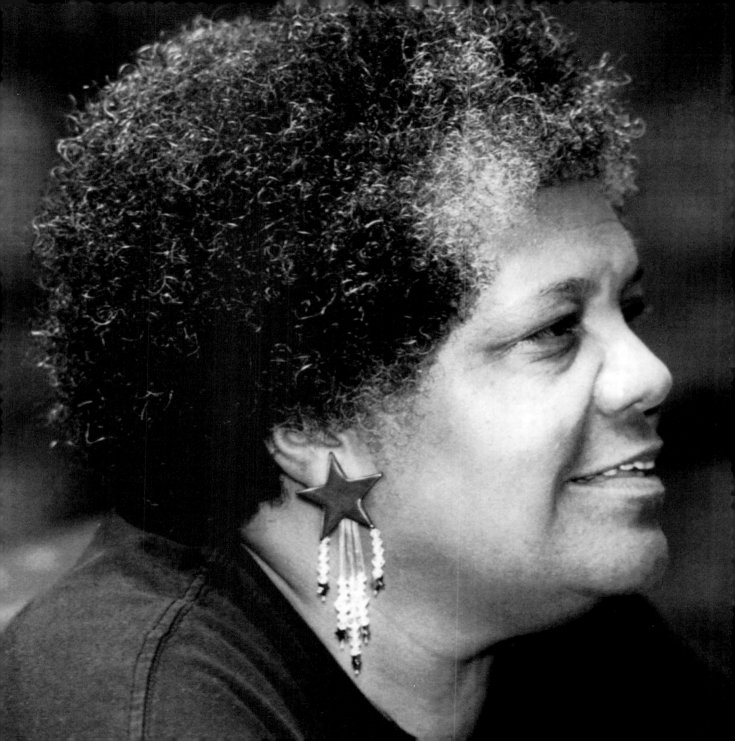

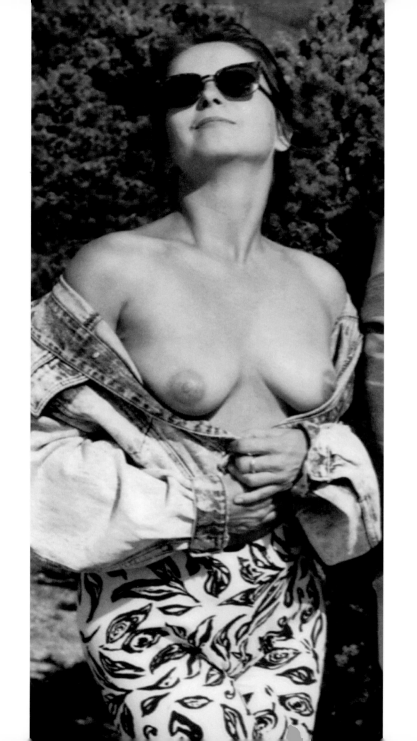

BEAUTY IS MINE BECAUSE

cancer could not break my spirit,
scars could not mutilate my body,
loss could not diminish my joy,
and fear could not prevent me from being in love.

Because morphine could not erase my good memories,
pain could not hamper my activities,
tomoxifen could not dry up my juices,
and a 50/50 chance for survival could not preoccupy my mind.

Because I remember that the time of death is uncertain, and in that knowing
the duality of hope and fear ceases to exist.

Sabina
Santa Fe, New Mexico

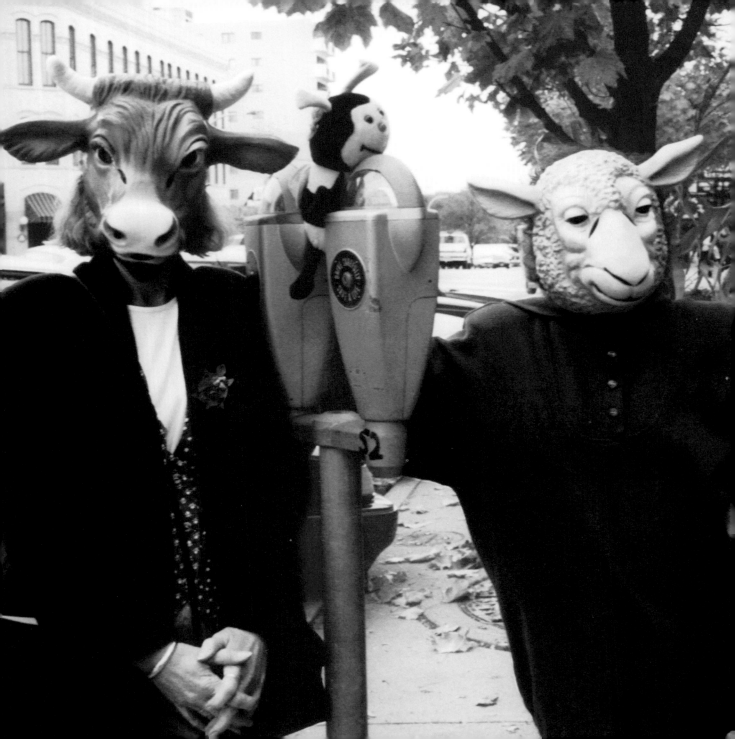

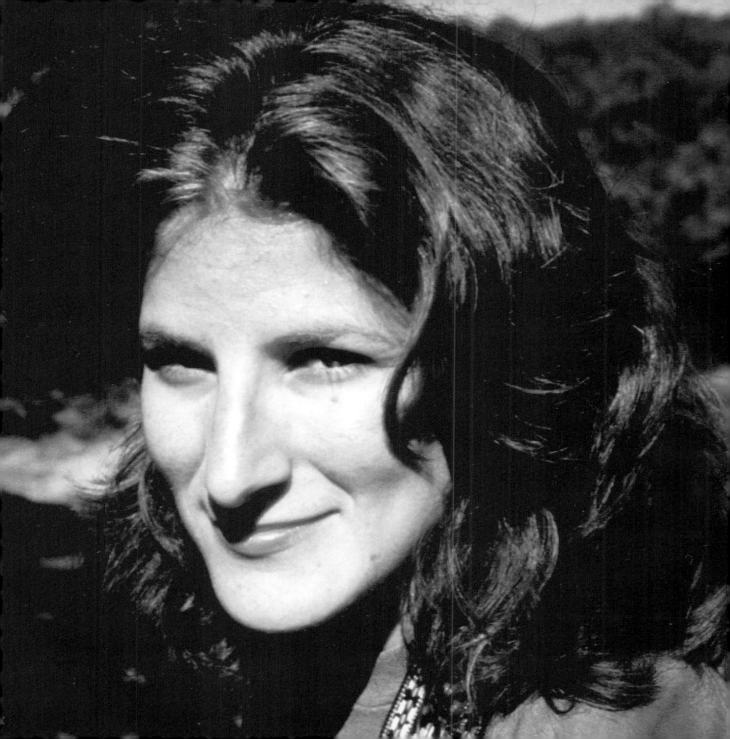

TODAY MY BEAUTY SHINES

because I brought my past into the present by undertaking a pilgrimage. I journeyed back to a place of great significance, a place where I stood in haunting loneliness 45 years earlier. As I ventured, I encountered people and spirits from my past. I faced them all with the peace, joy, and composure of a 64-year-old woman who has learned the meaning of resolution. Today, with despair and disillusion lifted, I stood before the awesome beauty of the Grand Tetons and soaked it in.

Rosalyn
St. Joseph, Michigan

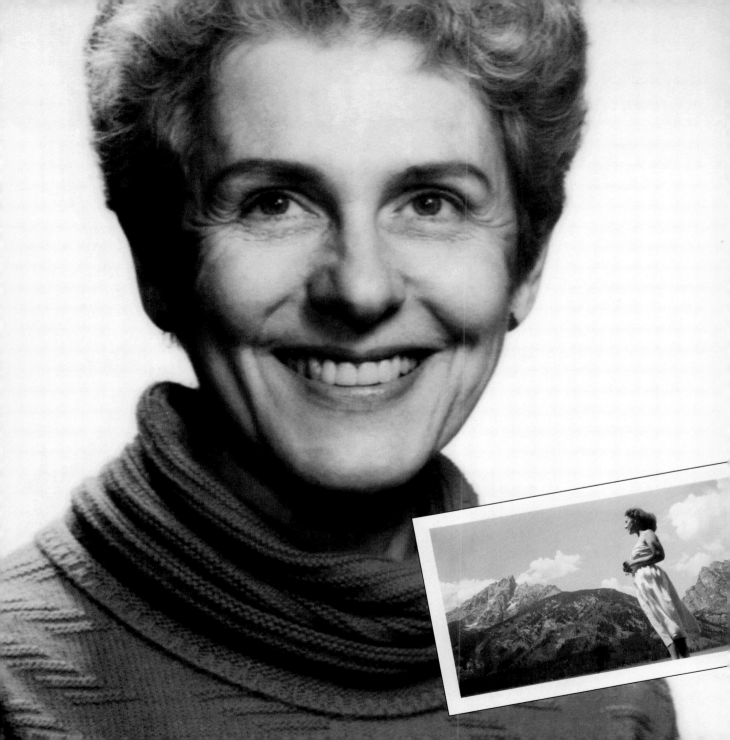

I MADE A CHOICE

that left me without the marriage I had dreamed of. I thought my marriage would shine like the spokes of a young girl's new two-wheeler. But before I could feel the joys of my dream, he hurt me.

So I left to find a shiny new life of my own. My beauty lies in knowing that I was worthy of the happiness I had dreamed of. I found it inside of me.

Lynae
Pasadena, California

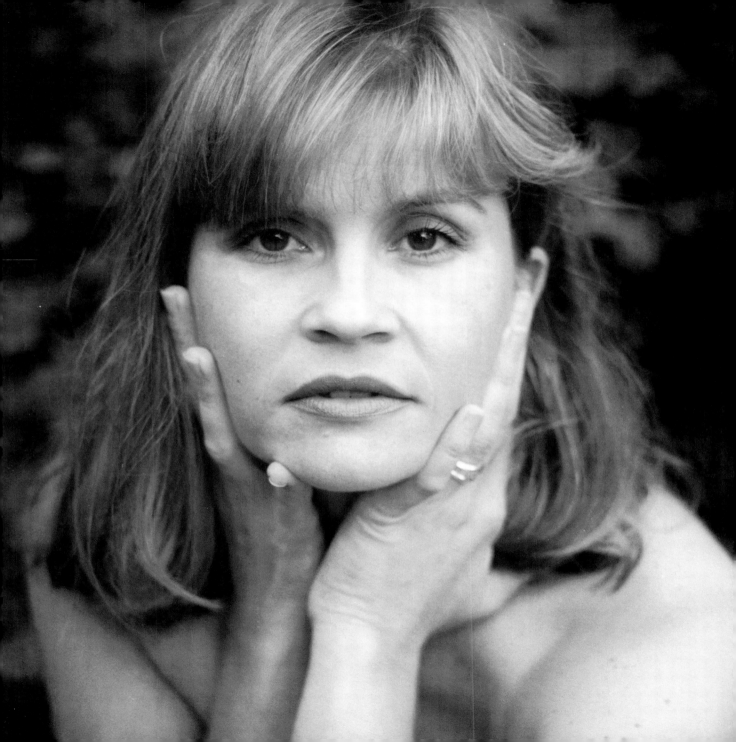

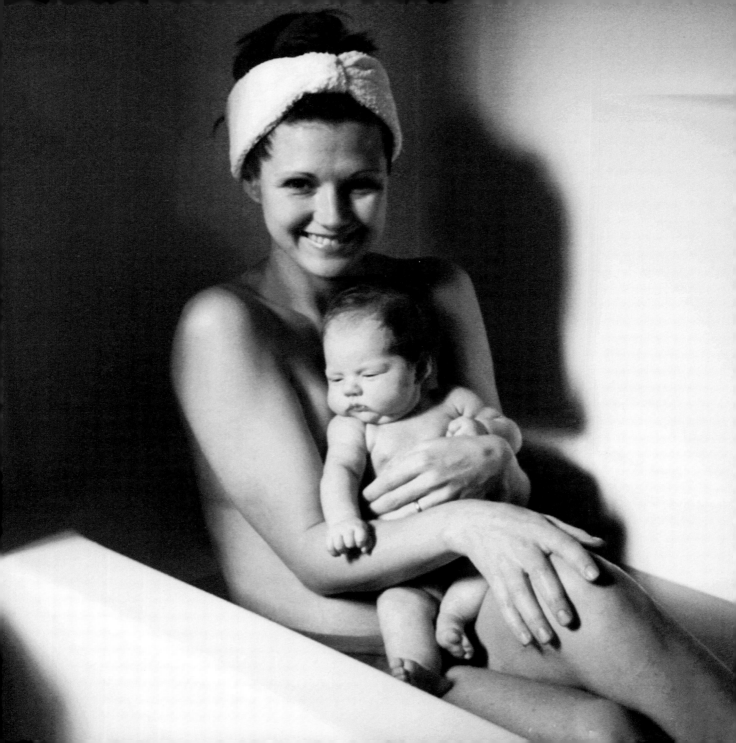

BEING BEAUTIFUL IS MY JOB,

and one I am well paid for. Since age 24, I have been a model and actress with enviable success. My beauty, however, eluded me until the roles changed from temptress to mom.

Forty years old and pregnant, with swollen belly and varicose veins, I am now seeing my beauty. I blissfully share the findings of my 3-year-old discovering her world. In my return to knee level, I see life with a rekindled passion.

I treasure this gift. It is my way of seeing that is my beauty.

Dorothy with her daughter, Jacqueline
Sherman Oaks, California

MY BEAUTY IS LIKE THUNDERING STALLIONS

galloping across grassy meadows, free and untamed.

My beauty extends over mountains, oceans, seas, over the land, for there are no boundaries to it.

My beauty contains the light of the world. The spirit of love and goodness shines within me like the glowing lava, which overflows, gracing me.

I am a living account of all the beautiful women who have walked, head high, into the deadly flames of oppression—women who spilled their tears, their sweat, and their blood upon the fires so that others could follow without being burned as badly.

Rosie
Atlanta, Georgia

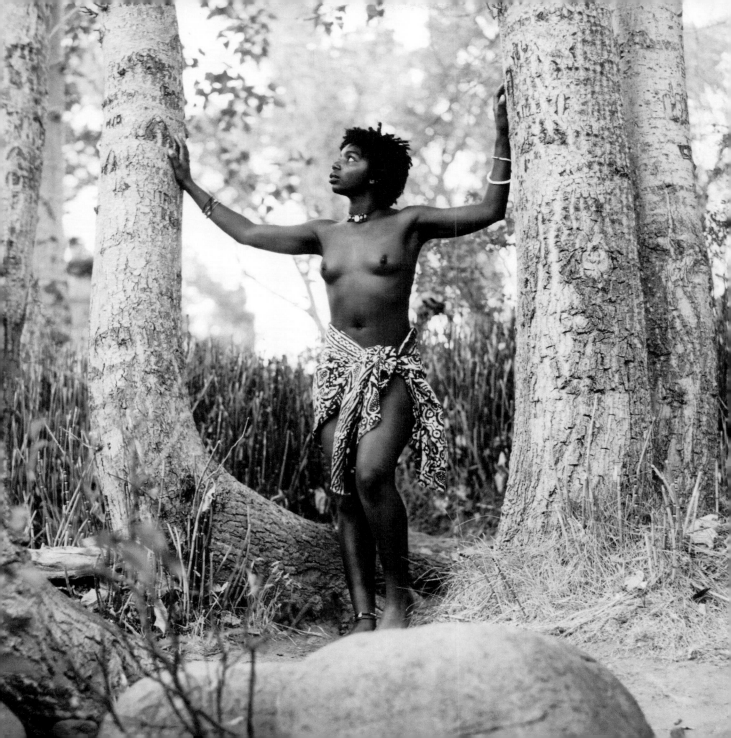

I MADE A DECISION ON MY 50TH BIRTHDAY

that defines my beauty. Looking back at the shards of what was then my mirror, I saw a plain, brown, hungry mouse trying for glamorous cathood scurrying on a treadmill, literally trying to work my tush off. On that day I asked myself, why? It was a question I could not answer.

I dropped my bags of costumes, curlers, and cosmetics, smashed my mirror with a spike-heeled boot, found a pen, and wrote: Being of sound mind (having just come to my senses), strong heart, and newly awakened spirit, from this day forward I will learn to say "No" to pain, paint, wire, starvation, and elastic. "No" to men who want a fold-out, pin-up, show-girl. "No" to women who want that kind of man. "No" to glamor. "Yes" to health. "Yes" to the natural beauty that I am.

Jo
San Antonio, Texas

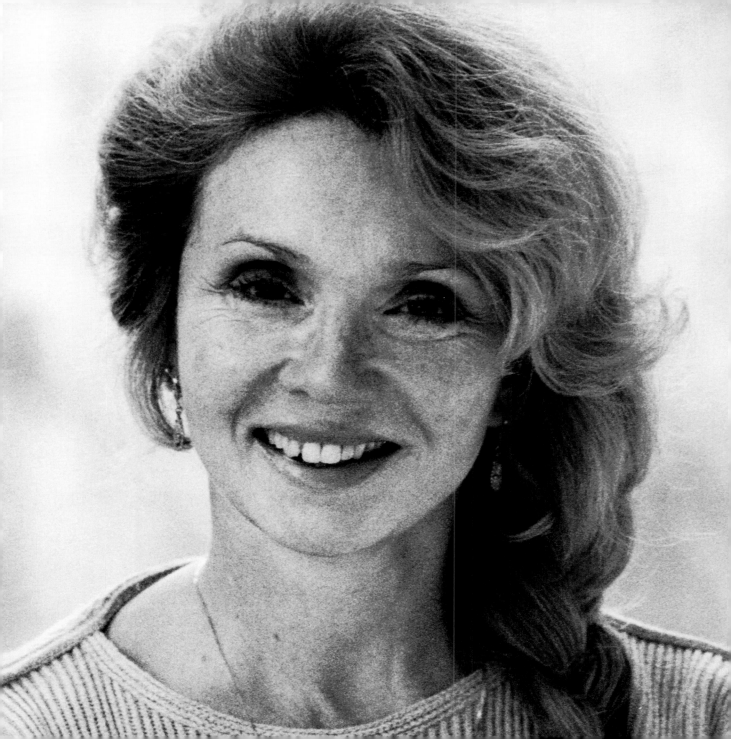

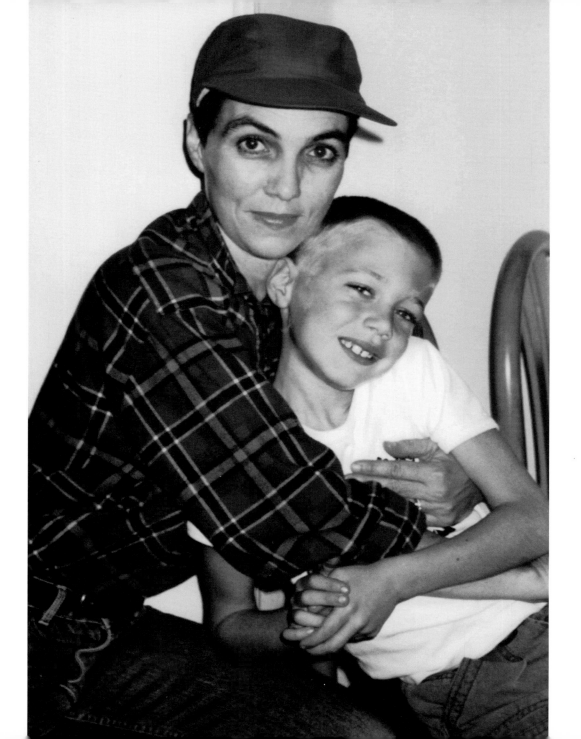

I WAS FEARFUL, HESITANT.

My hands shook as I packed my belongings on discharge day. I'd have to cover my head to avoid traumatizing the boys. I thought of Frankenstein every time I caught a glimpse of myself in the mirror.

One whole side of my face was pushed out grotesquely, and neat but vivid scars crossed from ear to ear, held together by dozens of mean-looking little staples. Purple and yellow bruises defined my temples and cheeks. This, in addition to newly healing burr holes, made my stubbly scalp look like someone's idea of a "Don't Wear Fur" campaign. Of course the kids would have questions, but did I need to scare them first?

After settling on my bed at home, the first thing my older son asked was what my head looked like under the scarf. Before I could answer, my 6-year-old snatched it off my head. I expected him to be repulsed by the scars and metal stuck in my scalp, but he simply said, "Oh cool. Mom's got a buzz," and cuddled into the crook of my arm. His mom was home and that was a beautiful thing to see.

Trish with her son, Alex
Northbrook, Illinois

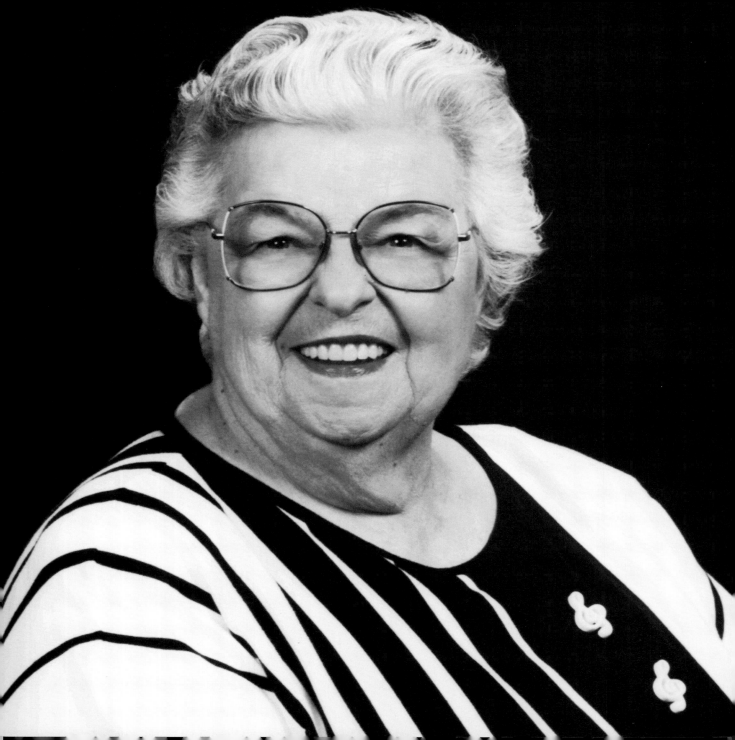

AS A CHILD OF THE DEPRESSION,

I knew things would improve; they did.

As a Navy W.A.V.E., I hoped for a better tomorrow; it arrived.

As a wife and mother, I knew life would be forever changing; it is.

As a single parent, raising two sons, I prayed for a new life partner; he arrived and we had 16 glorious years together before his death.

As an inveterate questioner and seeker, I wanted a college degree; I got it at age 54.

As a widow, I've learned contentment, and today

I respect my body and accept obesity as my lot.

At age 71 I can look back on my life and know
that God has been good to this big, beautiful woman.

Ollie
Palm Springs, California

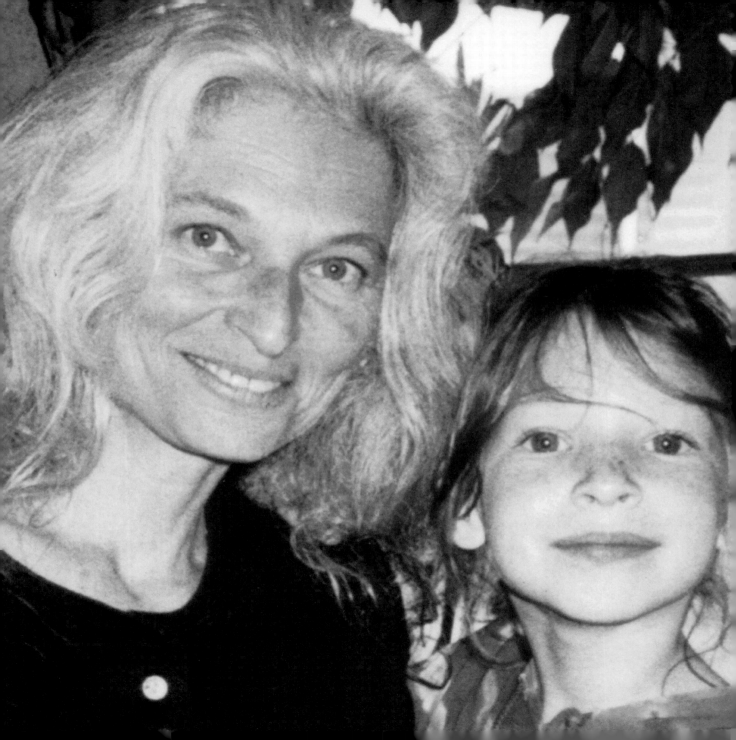

WHEN YOU FIRST SEE ME—

middle-aged, with the courage to judge worn on my face and the silver hair, my crown of wisdom—standing next to the maiden, I look more like the crone than the mother. Once my daughters asked me to dye my hair. "Why?" I asked. "To look younger," they replied. In my world, looking younger has no reward. It has taken me years to gain credibility with my words. Now it also comes with my appearance. Why would I want to change that?

Jeannine Parvati with
her daughter, Halley Sophia
Junction, Utah

I SHAVE MY HAIR

for I am not you as you are not I
I shave my hair for I am no better than you as you are no better than I
I shave my hair for the thousand moments where I am
    judged as woman
    judged as long flowing tresses breast and ass
    condemned as silent not following the groove freak
    condemned as a label that a stranger slaps upon my being
    tortured as a woman
    tortured as a human
I rid myself of the physical notability in hopes
    that you may view the inner beauty and pain and breath
I rid myself in hopes that you may rid yourself of the assumptions
I rid myself so you may feel my humanness
I expose myself dreaming that you may do the same
I expose myself and pray.

Christina
Binghamton, New York

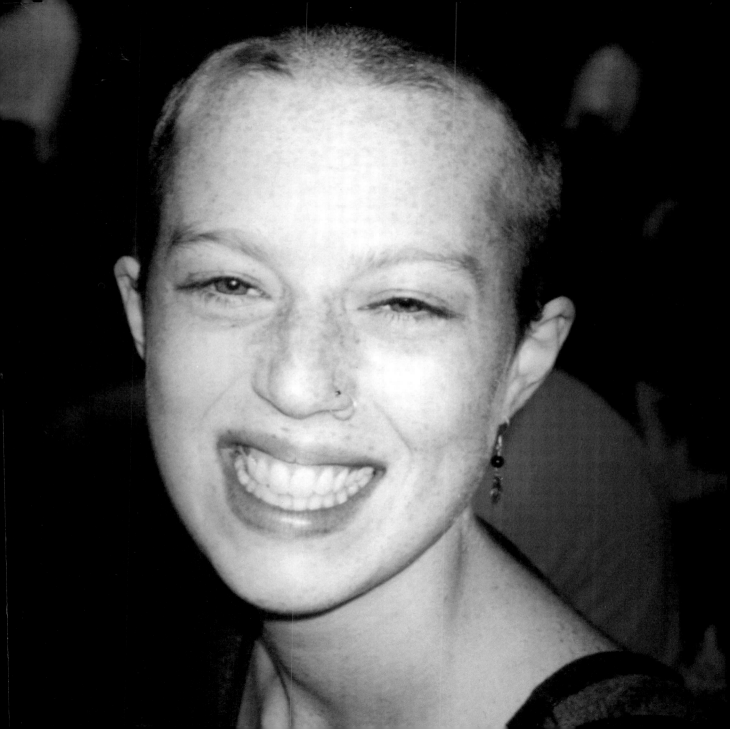